THE UN-UNCONSCIOUS OF MR. PSYCHIATRIST

By

Dr. Mohammad Reza Sargolzaee

Copyright © 2022 by Dr. Mohammad Reza Sargolzaee

All rights reserved. No part of this publication may be reproduced, stored, or transmitted in any form or by any means, electronic, mechanical, photocopying, recording, scanning, or otherwise without written permission from the publisher. It is illegal to copy this book, post it to a website, or distribute it by any other means without permission.

TABLE OF CONTENTS

Dedication	V
Acknowledgment	VI
Translator's Note	VII
Introduction	VIII
Therapeutic Deadlock	XI
Chapter One-Equation of Two Unknowns	1
Chapter Two-The Land of Strangers	5
Chapter Three-Super Ego	9
Chapter Four- The Oak Tree café	14
Chapter Five- Rene Descartes	18
Chapter Six-The Rabbit and The Eagle	22
Chapter Seven- Norwegian Wood	27
Chapter Eight- The Fratricide	33
Chapter Nine- The Farewell Waltz	40
Federal Republic of Puppets	47
Chapter One-Conflict	48
Chapter Two-Family Size Soda	53
Chapter Three- The Pragmatist	55
Chapter Four- Richard Bandler	58
Chapter Six- Theodora	62
Chapter Seven- The Oedipus	66
Chapter Eight- Christian Bobin	69
Chapter Nine-A Father's Signature	71
Chapter Ten- Socrates	73
Chapter Eleven-Departure	75
Nightmares of a postmodern Shaman	76
Chapter One-The Sacred Throne	77

Chapter Two-The Shaman	82
Chapter Three-The Safety Net	87
Chapter Four- The Purgatory	89
Chapter Five- Che Guevara	93
Chapter Six-Dream Analysis	97
Chapter Seven-Rubber Band	100
Chapter Eight- Damascus	102
Chapter Nine-The Aftermath	105
About the Author	107

Dedication

Dedicated to those who were just a number in the statistics,
but for freedom and to us,
They were boys, girls,
They were sisters, brothers,
They were our friends.

Acknowledgment

Thanks, Negar, for giving birth to the book for the English-speaking audience.

Special thanks to my editor, Tina, for her contributions to the English version.

Translator's Note

The book you are reading is the lived experience of Dr. Mohammad Reza Sargolzaee, a psychiatrist and social psychology's researcher in Iran, it is a book with a personal theme, which according to his words has been subjected to Regime's censorship several times as well as self-censorship, although maybe the revisions and self-censorships have made the book more mature.

The reason why I chose this book was that a large part of his writings are quotations of the thoughts of thinkers who were accepted at the time of writing the book by himself and it is very informative and educational book in this respect.

I highly value the thought and knowledge of Dr. Sargolzaee and the main reason for my devotion was when he announced a call for criticism review for his books so that in the next editions of his books, his books would be published with criticism review, and I think this is a unique and it was valuable that distinguishes him and his thoughtfulness.

Negar khaiyat kolkari

Introduction

Why am I telling this story?

A friend texted and asked me to name the most influential book of my life. His question, 'the most influential book,' seemed a deep and heavy phrase, making it difficult to answer. Of course, naming a book that changed the course of my life requires an inner journey, so here I go!

In the third grade of primary school, my parents gave me a book, *'Heroic kid,'* written by Ali Vafi. The story depicted an Egyptian child named Saeed. The author claimed that the city of Port Said in Egypt was named in his honour. The book narrated the story of the nationalization of the Suez Canal under the command of Gamal Abdel Nasser and the invasion of foreign forces into Egypt. Saeed, the protagonist, who was my age at the time, risked his life in a dangerous operation to destroy the military targets of the invading forces. This book contributed to a part of my belief system, and courage became one of the meaningful values of my life.

When I reached the fourth grade, I read Victor Hugo's *'Les Misérables.'* A year later, *'One Peach, A Thousand Peaches,' 'Twenty-four hours between sleep and waking,'* and *'Fable of Love'* by Samad Behrangi. Those stories sharpened my mind to the subject of poverty and discrimination, turning the justice into a noble pursuit that should be stood up for with bravery. Nearly a decade later, perhaps around eighteen, the books *'Abuzar, the theist socialist'* by Abdul Hamid Jodeh al-Sahar, which were translated and edited by Dr. Shariati, and the books *'Bread and Wine'* and *'Seeds under the Snow'* by Ignazio Silone, the Italian activist and author, cemented the impact of those childhood books in me.

In the first grade of middle school, Jalal Al Ahmad's book *'Noon Wal Qalam'* influenced me in such a way that I wrote the first story of my life replicating his style and presented it to my literature teacher Mrs. Amir Rezaei. Impressed by the writing, she predicted that one day, I would become a writer.

During high school, Farid al-Din Attar's *'Tazkar-ul-Awliya'* dragged me into Sufism. A decade later, the collection of Paulo Coelho's books with the unique translation of Dr. Arash Hijazi revived that disposition in me. This time, I went to Maulana's *'Masnavi'* and wandered in its chapters for years. If my belief system had not been shaken by a seven-magnitude earthquake and the destruction of that inner world had not led me to a 'Copernican revolution,' I might have still believed in those stories. Do you see? The story of our lives is shaped by stories. In my case, my early childhood was shaped by the tales of bravery, courage, and Sufism.

Neuroscience studies suggest that the hemispheres of the brain have different functions. What we normally call logical function (i.e, information analysis, mathematical logic, and language), are controlled by the left hemisphere, while artistic perception, including aesthetics, poetry, and music, is handled by the right hemisphere of our brain. Essentially, the right hemisphere deals with the functions that create emotions. The power of art resides here. Evidently, many of our decisions are not driven by rational thinking and sound financial assessment, but they are formulated by our emotions.

Almost every smoker is aware of its harm, but they *like* smoking! Arthur Asa Berger, a professor of communication at the University of San Francisco, considers smoking a *ritual*, and a ritual is nothing more than portraying a story. In the words of Jonathan Gotshall, a man is a storytelling animal. As such, even smoking has a story. Although, Sigmund Freud was also correct. 'Sometimes a fag is just a fag!'

Many risky behaviours and toxic relationships continue only on the basis of internal narratives. For the same reason, the Swiss-English philosopher, Alain de Botton, has written several philosophical love stories to critique the romanticism that leads to tension and failure in relationships. By providing logical information to people, we communicate with half of their brains, without targeting the issues that have a strong emotional basis. With stories, our entire nervous system is involved, impacting our emotional motivation and decisions.

Therefore, the counsellor or therapist, who is supposed to resolve emotional issues, has no choice but to transform into an artist to be able to address the right hemisphere of the brain. By 'an artist,' I don't imply that this person should officially attend art courses or pursue an artistic career but mastering a way with words or behaviour to touch the emotions of their clients.

Milton Erickson, the American hypnotherapist and psychiatrist was such a person. He used gestures and tones to tell stories in such a way that his clients were 'fascinated' by his words. Later, Erickson coined a name for this fascination and called it 'medical hypnosis.' Perhaps the most applicable art in psychotherapy is the art of storytelling since it can be implemented in almost any environment with minimal resources. I believe that the secret to the long-lasting religious scriptures, such as *the Old and the New Testament*, the *Qur'an*, and Rumi's *Masnavi*, also lies in their artful storytelling.

Dr. Mohammad Reza Sargolzaee - Psychiatrist

March 2021

Therapeutic Deadlock

Chapter One-Equation of Two Unknowns

Most of the time, I think something is wrong, a piece of the puzzle is missing, and this scenario is flawed. We're stuck in a vicious cycle; when we try to fix it, it gets worse, and if we leave it alone, it also gets worse again.

-Do you drink your coffee with creamer?

-Thank you, black is fine.

-Sugar?

-No thank you, I have diabetes, no sugar please...

-I also have glucose-free sweetener in my drawer.

-No, no. Thank you. I like it bitter.

-Well, go ahead, I'm listening.

-Yes, so I was saying that life is a complicated and unsolvable puzzle, like an equation with two unknowns, but one side of the equation has not been given to you. It's like they're forcing you to solve it like a puzzle that they have taken a few pieces out, asking you to put it together.

- Who forced you to pick it? Who said you should solve any equation? Just live your life.

-I Can't. It's not possible at all. Is it possible to live without knowing where we came from, why we're here, and where we're going? But let's see the other side of the picture. Every moment in life, we are faced with a mystery. Let me give you an example. When I was a child, the TV showed a movie. Sadly, I cannot recall its name, but it went like this, some people had received an invitation from an unknown person to stay in a villa in the middle of an island for a few days. They were supposed to be at a certain place on the beach on a specific day and time, and a boat was waiting for them. When they all reached the boat, they all had one question, who was the host?

Surprisingly, the Captain didn't know either. He had also taken money from an unknown person and didn't know anything except that he had to take some people to an island. Now, put yourself in the place of one of those guests. You enter the island and go to the villa. The servants and the other guests warmly welcome you, but they know nothing about the host and his purpose of calling random people to the island. They were all hired through a letter and received orders and payments in the mail.

Well, once you are on the Island, you drink coffee and get to know other guests. You may decide to take a walk to the beach with one of the guests you like the most. Let's see if you can forget who invited you to the island and why, and live your life regardless of all these questions. Could you? I wonder if anyone could.

- Your coffee is getting cold.

-Thanks a lot!

-Can you tell me a bit about your life instead of talking in general terms and giving examples? Like I want to know about your career, your family, and a little about your upbringing.

-Sure. I know that if we want to reach a conclusion, I should tell you about my problem, and you should tell me what to do. But to be honest, what I said earlier is the reality of my life. I mean, it's not like I have a life apart from these, to which I could return, and close the door to these chaotic thoughts.

You said job... Let me start with my job. Well, when I'm sitting in my bookstore, someone comes to me and wants to buy a book for his friend's birthday, he asks for a recommendation, and I face the same struggles in life again. Let's say, I'm reading Silone's *'Bread and Wine'* for the third time.

I would like to recommend this book to him. However, the minute I would think of doing it, hundreds of questions would hit my brain. I ask myself, 'Are you sure this book is worth it? What impact did this book have on your life? The thesis of socialism without a party, Christianity without a church by Silone made you unable to survive within the framework of any party or church. Are you having a great time now that you have broken free of these frameworks? But isn't that the reason for your confusion and indecision? If you could trust the Central Council of the Party or the Council of Cardinals of the Church, wouldn't your life be much easier? You were at ease. They would tell you if you should participate in the elections or not, and if you were going to participate, they tell you who you should vote for. They used to tell you all the right and wrong things, and if you had followed that, you would have been living your life without worrying about the choices. You used to do as you were told, and you didn't go to the forbidden places.'

Well, when these thoughts cross my mind, I refrain from recommending *'Bread and Wine'* to my client. It's not better than nonsensical self-help books like *'Fall in love in 21 days'*, *'How to love everyone?'* or *'Four weeks to become a millionaire.'* When I'm about to hand one of these books to a customer, a voice in my head says, 'Is that in line with your cultural mission? Don't you think that most of the troubles of human beings are because they're too self absorbed? How to have more fun, how to make more money, and how to impress others? Don't you think it's necessary to offer these people some real questions? Instead of 'Why am I not making more money?' they should ask, 'why should we lie to each other?' If not, why did you become a book seller if you weren't to inflict pain and social awareness in people? You could have opened a flower shop or an ice cream parlor.'

Do you see? it's not that easy. I want to live my life, but how can I live with these thoughts? Tell me, if you were me, which book had you recommended to the customer and why?

-Well, I think your mind is too busy with right and wrong. Maybe you had strict parents who constantly scolded you for doing the wrong things. Sometimes such type of parents push their children to get involved in the complexity of right and wrong for the rest of their lives. And when this happens, children are afraid to make the wrong choice. It's as if they're afraid that their dads or moms will yell at them with that terrible frown, with that look, and with that wise tone, 'So, was it the right thing? Aren't you ashamed of yourself?'

-Maybe so. Well, my parents wanted us to study and be polite. For example, talk to elders with respect and greet them. I don't know, maybe I don't remember well, but I don't think they were that strict. In our house, no one ever forced me to pray, although everyone did. At the same time, if I had learned F words from the kids at the school and repeated them at home, they would have been very upset with me. Of course, all this did not stop me from swearing when I was angry. Honestly, I can't blame my parents, but if you think that accepting this idea will make me feel better, I'm ready to accept it.

-Alright! Your time's up, we'll talk about it more in the next session.

Chapter Two-The Land of Strangers

I've been thinking about your words for the past few days. That my parents might have caused my spiritual or philosophical concerns or whatever you want to call it. But I cannot agree with your opinion. Honestly, the more I reviewed my life, the more I saw that more than my family, I was influenced by books, movies, stories, teachers, and my friends. Let me give you an example,

As far as I remember, there wasn't much expression of love in our home.

When my parents were in a good mood, their relationship was friendly, not romantic. I don't remember them ever saying 'Dear' to each other; let alone 'My love.' Despite the unromantic environment, I started falling in love early in life. I think the first time I fell in love; I must have been 8 years old. It was in the second grade of primary school. At a party, I had spoken a few words to a girl about my age, her name was 'Homa.' She wasn't beautiful at all. She was not ugly, though. But I mean, it wasn't like I fell in love with her looks. It was just an arbitrary attraction that I had developed within seconds of session her. Can you believe that I though about 'Homa' for months, maybe even years. When I went to a fun place, I missed her by my side. At that age! Just think about it!

Is it normal? When I was in the fourth year of primary school, a girl from our family fell in love with me. I liked her too, but I didn't fall in love with her. At that age, I could tell the difference between liking and love! I knew that I liked her, but she was in love with me. After that, I fell in love again at twelve or thirteen. I was in love with one of the girls in the neighbourhood, whose name was

'Mina.' I used to think about her all day. I went to the alley with different excuses, so I could pass by her house to just stare at its door! Well, not all these love stories were beautiful, some hold a lot of nostalgia.

The point is, if we assume that falling in love can be learned, I did not learn it in our home. Not only did my parents not have a romantic attitude, but as far as I can remember, most of our relatives were kind of people who thought more about marriage and settling down than love.

I think that if I had learned love from somewhere, it was not my home. Maybe it was from movies. I had watched several of those Persian films that were popular at that time. Similarly, there were 7-8 Hindi movies, with the common themes of romance, but those movies didn't have a deep impact on me. I mean, the thought of watching romantic movies never excited me. I was never ready to watch one of these movies instead of *'Bruce Lee,'* *'The Six Million Dollar Man,'* and other action movies.

I preferred gangster and cowboy movies, especially those involving pirates. Even comedy movies interested me more than romantic movies. When I was eleven or twelve years old, I was reading Victor Hugo's novel *'Les Misérables.'* As much as 'Jean Valjean,' the powerful and kind-hearted prisoner was attractive to me, the romantic scenes of Cosette and Marius seemed spoiled and unbelievable. It was only after falling in love multiple times that I realized only a romantic story of my type appeals to me.

I mentioned my type of love because I feel that loving has different colours; Blue love is different from red love, and pink love is different from heavenly love.

-What colour is your love?

-Fortunately, or not, I don't know. I can't choose a particular colour and stick to it for the rest of my life. But if it comes to my mind, I will tell you.

Basically, the point I want to make is that, growing up, the outside events affected me more than the events inside our home. Plus, it seems that there's something or things inside me that could not be learned. It's like I had them from within. Only when I encounter their equivalents in the outside world, I feel familiar and connected with it. For example, I first experienced love in myself, then I found examples of it manifested in stories. That was a relief.

-Why a relief?

Yes, I really breathed a sigh of relief. When I found love outside myself, I had the same feelings a native Persian living in a foreign country would feel after session someone who speaks Farsi. You know, doctor, if no one else has an experience and only you have that experience, you tend to feel very alienated. Imagine that you see a person in your house that no one else can see, and when you talk about him or her, everyone looks confused as if you are crazy. Think how hard it is! But how relieved you will be when another person can see that creature.

When I read the love of Santiago and Fatima in *'The Alchemist'* by Paulo Coelho, or when I read the poems of the late Nader Ebrahimi in *'Ibn Attarih'* and *'Abol al-Mashaghel,'* or even when I perceive the confusion of young people in the movie *'Under the Moonlight,'* I felt that I was not alone. I breathed a sigh of relief. Sometimes, at times like this, I start to cry as if I am bursting with loneliness.

-Do you cry a lot?

-No, not much. I rarely cry, maybe once every few months. I remember crying while watching Hatami Kia's movie 'Glass Agency.' In that scene where 'Haj Kazem' opens his wife Fatima's letter and sees his shirt and license plate that she left for him, I cried a lot. The more I thought that Fatima understood and felt Haj Kazem's inexplicable madness, the more I cried.

Are you tired, doctor?

-No, no, why did you think I'm tired?! I'm listening intently.

-Your eyes look tired and red, and you yawned a few times. I'm sorry, I didn't mean to be rude. All I'm suggesting is if you're tired, we can finish a little earlier today.

-It's fine. Would you like to finish the session early? Did the things you speak of exhausted you?

-No, but honestly, you know what I say is very important to me. I put a lot of pressure and force on myself to come here and talk. And that's why I don't want you to listen to me impatiently. Of course, I too feel tired, but the fact that I asked was not really because I wanted to finish early, I wanted your attention. I want your mind to be clear and sharp when I speak, so you can fully understand me.

-You force yourself to come here? How?

-The truth is, I can't really be hopeful that some talking will solve my problems. Regardless, I decided to exhaust all the avenues, but I still didn't come here with much hope. Forgive me, I don't intend to insult you and question your expertise, just want to be honest. Anyway, I'm paying for something that I don't even expect to work out, and this is not cheap, at least for me.

I'm sorry, I didn't mean to say these things, just wanted to make sure you're not too tired. I can imagine it's not easy to sit for 4-5 hours and listen to people like me.

-Well, maybe you're right, I honestly can't say I don't feel tired at all. Would you like to have some Nescafe?

-Sure. Thank you very much!

-No creamer and no sugar. See? I remember every word; you're diabetic and you prefer bitter coffee!

Chapter Three-Super Ego

So, where do we start? It's been a long while since our last session.

-Are you asking, or should I speak again?

-Please continue. I think you were talking about your love life in the previous session.

-Well, not exactly. I intended to mention more than love. I was giving you a few examples as to why my family did not influence me that much. I think I was successful in explaining how many words from many people had influenced my thoughts and feelings more than my parents. Our time was short, or else I would've told you that there was something in me that could not be learned. It happened to me. I don't know where it came from, but I experienced it within myself before anyone told me anything about them. Do you still think I should look for the root of my issues in my parents' behaviour?

-I don't insist. Maybe we can talk more about it another time. Tell me, do you still fall in love?

-That's a complicated question! Honestly, I don't have a one-word answer for it. One day my son asked, 'Dad, do we only fall in love once?' And I answered that it depends on the individual. Some people never fall in love, and they don't experience love, neither do they talk about it. Then there are people who talk about love but never experience it.

In my perspective, some fall in love only once, some fall in love many times, and some are always in love, even when they don't have a lover. It's like their lover is gone or has not showed up yet, anyway, they're always in love.

-Okay, if that's the case, which category are you?

-Unfortunately, I think I'm one of those who fall in love many times!

-Unfortunately? Why do you think it's unfortunate to fall in love multiple times?

-I said unfortunately, because many times there is a 'No Entry' sign posted in front of the alley of love.

-Who installed that sign? Your mom and dad? Or the movies you watched and the stories you read?

-Do you think there is no such sign?

-Please answer my question. It would be much easier if we understand who posted that sign in your head? Was it you mom and dad? Or was it the movies you watched and the stories you read?

-All of them, Doctor. All of them! My parents, movies, stories, history, philosophy, literature, religion, culture, education; all of them posted the 'No Entry' sign in my head. Doctor, do you really believe there's no such thing as 'forbidden love' and all kinds of love are acceptable?

-I never said anything like that. I just wanted to know where your 'forbidden love' sign came from. I wanted to better understand its origin. Something to think about.

-Yes, I would think about it because that's all I think about most of the times. If you don't mind, let me explain to you through an example.

-Yeah sure, go ahead!

-Look, when a boy and girl, both belonging to respectable and supportive families meet each other and spend some fun time together, they develop attraction towards each other. The couple then decide to call this feeling 'love' and tell their families about each other. The families think their children are in love and investigate this matter. Only when they realize the person that their child loves and the person's family has a similar lifestyle to them, they come to this conclusion that the other party can be trusted.

After the necessary arrangements, this love meets the traditional, religious, and legal requirements, and there is no obstacles in reaching their ultimate destination – marriage. This is a kind of love. Now, fifteen years into the marriage of this couple, the feeling they once identified as love has slowly changed, it has evaporated in the thin air or matured or become infected.

It's highly possible that something has happened to them due to which they're no longer in love. I feel that this love is not the love they had perceived in the beginning of their relationship. That feeling may be something in the middle, but whatever that feeling is, it's not love. If you want to call it love, call it love, but they're aware that this is something other than the initial love.

-So, what's wrong? Life is in motion; nothing remains constant, everything's changing. What do you think is wrong in here?

-You're right. I know that life is ever changing, but the topic of my discussion is not that the feeling should not change. What I want to imagine is fifteen years after this marriage, one person in the marriage experiences the same intense feeling they had experienced years ago or something similar with another person – a completely different being!

-Okay, and?

-Okay? Doctor, imagine it's me after fifteen years of marriage, with two children and a life that's seemingly perfect from the point of view of an outside observer.

I've such an experience. A lady comes to our bookstore three times in a row, and the fourth time she visits, I feel like I'm going to lose myself. I'm clumsy and agitated , wanting our chats to be longer, so she stays longer, and then I notice that she has also stayed more than what's necessary to wonder around in a bookshop.

-Then?

-Well, then I see that I'm thinking about her a lot. I'm living in an illusion, far away from reality. When I hear a romantic song, I remember her, and when I hold 'Hafiz' in my hand, I want to ask him about our love (A type of fortune telling by using the poems - Translator).

-And then?

- Then my wife feels that I've changed. She feels that I'm not the same person anymore. She feels that I've become restless and impatient and that I am hiding something from her. This, in turn, makes her restless and nervous because she can't find any reason for that feeling. At present, she's whinging about everything. She complains about stuff, and every day she has pain somewhere in her body.

-And how does this make you feel?

-It feels like I'm bearing a heavy crushing pressure. I feel like crashing under a cloud of my own desires and her expectations. What should I do? I share her pain. I blame myself and feel guilty.

-You feel guilty?

-Yes, doctor. I feel guilty because...

-Okay, so did you feel guilty when you were a child?

-When I was a child... Umm. I don't remember accurately. Maybe I felt guilty once or twice, but I'm not quite sure. I had a happy childhood. Everything was fun and I think I enjoyed it a lot, because I like everything that reminds me of my childhood – the city where I grew up, the neighbourhood, the songs, the movies, and those old cartoons... I don't think I felt much guilt as a child, even if I did, it wasn't so much that I remember. Doctor, my parents were not familiar with 'Freud,' but they didn't burden my 'super ego' that much. Believe me, this has nothing to do with my childhood. As a human being, I can't be indifferent to the impact I have on others.

-Why do you seem angry?

-We'll talk about it again in our next session. The time's up; it was nice talking to you.

Chapter Four- The Oak Tree café

Hello! Shall I start again?

-Hi! If you want to say something important, I'll listen. Otherwise, I'll start with a question, how about that?

-This sounds better. You ask, and I'll answer your questions.

-Is it okay if I smoke my pipe? Does the smell of tobacco bother you?

-No, no, that's fine. I'm okay with it.

-Thanks. Well, here's my first question, In the previous sessions, you talked about your problems in detail, so I now know what type of life you don't want. However, I'm still confused about the life you want. So, if you were to write the description of your life yourself, how exactly would you write it? In this session, I would like you to talk on this subject, so I can figure out what type of life you want for yourself.

-Well, that's a great question. Let me gather my thoughts for a while.

-I think you should think out loud. I don't want you to organize your thoughts. Speak as you think. It's more interesting and helpful to me. Let me hear your thoughts!

-Yes, yes, I got your point. I will definitely do so. First, I wish I wasn't so emotional. I wish I wasn't so sensitive. If so, I hadn't suffered so much. I think I had lived much easier. You know, Doctor, in my opinion, if I were a different person, there would be no need to change my life because my life was never a problem. The problem is me, myself. Let me give you an example. A few days ago, I was sitting in my friend's café. This place is my hangout, kind of a cozy corner to be alone with myself. Although the café belongs to one of my friends, he used my ideas to set it up. That's why I feel like home there.

-Could you explain a bit more?

-Sure. For example, the name of the café – he named it 'Oak Tree Café' at my suggestion. I don't know whether you've read '*1984*' by George Orwell or not.

-No, I haven't read it. I only read 'Animal Farm' by George Orwell. And that too was many years ago when I was in my late teens.

-In that book George Orwell writes about 'Oak Tree café,' a place where painters and musicians hang out and sitting there exposes one to arrest by the 'thought police.' In fact, it can be said that the hangout is for those who are still able to think, and their brains are more than a voice recorder and slogan player.

-Well, very interesting!

-Exactly. There's also another meaning to this name; usually owls make their nests in the oak tree, so I also meant that this cafe could be a hangout for owls.

-Owls? Wow! I'm surprised. It's said that owls are bad omen.

-No, doctor. The ominous legend of the owl is exclusive to this region. In the other places and countries, owls are wise birds, and forest animals turn to them whenever they face an unsolvable problem in their lives.

I think wisdom has something to do with loneliness. As long as a person is with other people, he's so immersed in the flow of life that he cannot look at life properly. He looks at the parts of life, but not at the big picture! I think we cannot understand our whole life by looking at some fragments of it. As German philosophers say, life is a 'gestalt' – a whole greater than the sum of its parts. Moreover, you cannot understand it by looking at the individual parts. It's like a puzzle that if you look at all the thousand pieces one by one, you can't picture the whole puzzle.

For you to understand the puzzle, the pieces must be arranged next to each other and in their place, and then you look at all the pieces, perceiving the entire picture. Life is like this, you can not understand it with an analytical view, you should look at it all at once and in one place. And for this, you must pull yourself out of the flow of life. That was what 'Buddha' and many others who wished to understand life did. Well, the owl is only a symbol of wisdom, and the oak tree is the place of the owl. People, out of the hoo-ha of life, alone but wise.

-Well, it seems like a compelling idea.

-Yes, Doctor. I was sitting in the Oak Tree Café holding a newspaper. The only interesting news for me was that of a violin duet that two sisters had performed. I was removing that piece from the newspaper to put it on my calendar when my friend (the cafe owner) sat next to me and started talking. He talked about his mother, who has cancer and told me that for a few days she has been in the hospital for radiology, tests, etc. Between his talks, he said that he has been travelling to and from the hospital for the past few days, and that made him realize we should be so grateful to God.

He said while in the hospital, he saw people who did not have money for their kid's medicine, people who begged to admit their child, but they were denied entry because they did not have enough money. With no money, the hospital staff shunned them. My friend said the depressing scenes in the hospital made him contemplate the way he was living his life. It instilled in him the habit of being thankful to God for the blessings he and his family were receiving. He told me that whenever he thought about the money he spends only on fast food every time he takes his children out, he thanked God that he's not in that awful situation.

-Okay, it's good that he's developed the power of showing gratitude.

-Yes, doctor. A devastated father and a tired worker begging for his child to be hospitalized had pushed my friend to thank God that he's not in that situation. However, not experiencing this scene myself and only hearing the description from my friend, since that day I felt miserable. I had this feeling constantly lingering in my head.

I cannot thank God by witnessing such scenes, I'm indebted to God! Why should there be such miseries in the divine system to make us understand how blessed we are? Why? I just looked at my friend who was thanking God, I couldn't answer him. In my heart, I was disgusted. I either had to remain silent or I had to shout, 'What kind of world is this? What kind of God is this? What kind of justice is this?' And I chose to remain silent.

Since the day in the café, I still feel sick. Maybe that child has finally been admitted to the hospital. Maybe he has recovered. Or that hard-working father is still thinking it's very normal that he doesn't have money and begging the receptionist to admit his son to the hospital. But me...

I can't stand it. I feel sick. My heart wants to explode, I want to scream at everyone, at myself, at my friend, at the receptionist, at the head of the hospital, the head of the government, the head of God! Doctor, I wish I wasn't so sensitive and emotional, and I could just have a cup of Latte at the Oak Tree and thank God like my friend did, for being able to take my children to a fancy restaurant that night.

I wish I could... Are you tired, doctor?

- No dear, I'm thinking.

-I think my time's up, right?

-Time? Oh, yes, that's right! I'll see you next week.

Chapter Five- Rene Descartes

In the previous session, you talked about that poor person who could not admit his child to the hospital. How much has it affected you? I think it might not be bad for us to revisit that memory and elaborate on it, right?

-Yes, of course, Doctor. Thank you for actually listening and thinking about my words.

-You're welcome. See, you're looking at the glass half empty. Each of us has experienced suffering somewhere in this life, but we had a lot of fun in some places as well. Even that poor man may have bagged more than you and me in his life.

You're just looking at that person's suffering. Maybe if you could access the child's life a week before, or a week after this scene, you will see that child playing with his friends with extreme joy and happiness. You will see how the child is healthy and is enjoying life. Now even if you focus on the suffering, you cannot still complain that the poor man or the sick child is a victim.

While this might not be the case here, generally speaking, our choices in our lives impact our future. How do you know if that poor man had made more effort and used more creativity in his life, the situation would not have been different? Aren't there a few people who start as workers and then become factory owners? If someone touches the fire, his hand will naturally burn and hurt. Now, if you remove the happy sequence from this series and only watch the suffering sequence, it is natural that you think this person is a victim of suffering. And you will inevitably sympathize with him, but if you remember that this person's current situation is influenced by his previous choices, then your feeling will be different.

-You are logically correct. It can be said that our life is affected by our choices – good and bad. As a result of good choices, we are proud of ourselves. Additionally, we ourselves are responsible for the pains we suffer.

Even if someone says that little children who do not have the choice in the suffering, disease, disability, paralysis, blindness, deafness, etc., they can find a convincing answer. For example, Hindus and some Buddhists believe that we're coming into this world again and again and we live a different life each time, and each of these lives is influenced by our past lives. So, when a person is born in a poor family, it might be because he had lived a lavish life as a rich man and violated the rights of the poor. Hence, in his new life as an impoverished person, he has come to pay for the things he did previously. Similarly, a child who was born blind may have been a cruel king or a cruel executioner in his previous life. Maybe he was the ruler or an ordinary man who caused the blindness of several people and is now being punished. These things can be true, Doctor! The beautiful hypothesis of 'reincarnation' has answers to all questions, it's a pity that it cannot be proven in any way. But for the same reason, it cannot be rejected either. Those who do not want to accept the Hindu reincarnation find other answers to this problem. They believe that our real life is our spiritual life and we did not come to this world to enjoy, we came to polish and upgrade our soul and the more we suffer, the purer and purer our soul becomes, so after seeing these people who suffer endlessly in this world, we should say, Blessed are those who suffer, they are closer to the Kingdom of God! Instead of doubting God's mercy and saying, O creator of the world, what is justice when you look and see so much suffering in the world?

I read these things in the books, so I can effortlessly weave all these hypotheses to convince people, but I'm suffering, I can't control my emotions. When I see a 5-year-old sitting on the corner of the sidewalk in the extreme cold of winter, wearing small clothes and putting the scale in front of him so that we can throw him a coin, I suffer. He can find his frozen palm in his pocket.

I can say that it's not my fault, nor God's fault, neither the glitch in the socio-political system, it's the addicts and irresponsible parents who are willing to exchange money for heroin and leave this innocent child out in the cold. I can say all this to myself, but in the next 3 hours, when having delicious food or wherever I go, I remember the face of that kid on the street still shivering in the cold, I feel disgusted and suffocated with hatred.

-Well, I think the way we think forms our feelings. It's strange that you can think rationally but still have annoying feelings.

-Unfortunately, logical thinking cannot control my emotions. Let me give you an example; Do you know 'Rene Descartes?'

-Descartes? Yes, yes, I've heard his name, French philosopher and mathematician and the founder of analytic geometry and all that, right?

-Yes, that's him. In addition to being a philosopher and a mathematician, Descartes also studied experimental sciences. Among his favourite works were autopsies and the dissection of animals.

-Wow! I didn't know.

-Yes, I read in a book that Descartes believed that animals lack 'intellect,' and since they don't have sense of intelligence, they don't have real feelings either. Do you know how this person dissected the poor animals? Without making them unconscious, while they were alive and screaming, he tied them and tore them to pieces. At that time, in response to those who objected to his work, he said that they really do not suffer! And when they said why are they screaming and shouting, he said if you crumple even a paper, it rustles. Just as the rustling of paper has nothing to do with its pain, the screaming of a cat has nothing to do with its pain, it's just a reaction, that's all!

-No! Have Descartes really done it?

-I can't say yes or no. I read this in a book but I cannot remember its name. Anyway, let's imagine such a cruelty has been done by someone.

-Okay?

-Yes, well, even if I'm convinced by the completely logical reasons of a great philosopher and scientist that the scream of this cat is like the rustling of paper and that animal is not really in pain, it still hurts me to hear its scream and noise, doctor. Believe me, despite the perfectly logical reasons, I would still suffer from their pain, I can't hear a cat scream and say, it's OK!

-I understand... I think I can't stand the screaming of a cat that is being dissected alive, too.

-Yes, doctor, I gave this example to say that it's not always possible to look differently and feel in a different way. We can't choose our feelings. If it were up to me to choose my feelings, I would have chosen never to experience 'compassion' and 'sympathy.' When I have performed my personal duty, why should I worry about something that is not my responsibility, and I have no authority to change it? I remember when I was a child, I cried after reading the books *'One peach and thousand peaches'* and *'Twenty-four hours between sleep and wakefulness'* by Samad Behrangi. I couldn't get the slum dwellers and poor people out of my head for months. I wish my heart could be made of stone or ice, so that my heart would not burn for anyone, and my heart would not ache for anyone. If that was the case, I would've lived so carefree, doctor... Would you help me?

-...

- Are you crying?

-Oh, no, no, this new tobacco is a bit heavy for me, it makes my eyes teary!

-Okay. And my time's over. I think it's time to leave.

Chapter Six-The Rabbit and The Eagle

SO, you said in the previous session that you cannot control your emotions. Right?

-That's right, Doctor, you asked me to think about an alternative scenario for this life, and I told you that if I wasn't so emotional, maybe life, as it is, was actually good. Rabbits intrude the farmlands in the village, and wolves eat baby rabbits. Really, why am I not upset when a rabbit chews on the grass, but an eagle squeezing a rabbit in its talons, makes me angry? It does not seem logical. I know, this is the cycle of life; we eat and are eaten. I read in a book by Alain de Botton, in which he quoted Schopenhauer, love is the same thing, almost in the same way. He considers the root of love to be 'the will to live.'

It means that it's just about reproduction, and that's it! Life wants to continue, and according to Darwin, natural selection needs diversity within species. Therefore, diverse and complementary genes must be preserved and developed in the genetic treasure of life. This causes people who carry complementary genes to be attracted to each other. The importance of this matter for life is not more than some turtles laying eggs or the mating season for the mountain goats! It seems completely logical, so doctor, all the romance novels in the world, Laila and Majnun, Anna Karenina, Doctor Zhivago, The Legend of Love, and… are Bullshit. They don't have much to do with reality.

The whole point is reproduction, and that's it. We are born into this world to eat, hatch, and die, and then our offspring will continue the cycle. It's all logical, doctor. Although it's bitter and ridiculous, I think it's scientific and logical. But knowing all this does not help me avoid love when I'm falling in love. You don't know how much I suffer. Those who know Schopenhauer and Darwin and never fall in love have no problem, those who know nothing about Schopenhauer and Darwin and fall in love have only one problem, and that's the pain of love. But doctor, I suffer the most. I know Schopenhauer and Darwin, and I still fall in love. I endure romantic longings and the burden of philosophical pressure, knowing well that all this game is just for reproduction. On the one hand, I'm emotional, and on the other hand, I smirk at my tender feelings. I'm confused whether the romantic tenderness is real or the wise scorn?

-Let me see, if you break this complex chain of thoughts and just experience life, what kind of life would you have?

-I can't fathom what you're suggesting.

-Look, when a feeling of longing or a tender feeling comes to you, you don't have to call it a romantic feeling, you don't have to take it to your analysing machine and see what Schopenhauer or Darwin or Freud or Plato had to say about it! So, let's assume that you are just a rabbit or an eagle, how would you live?

-Well, the rabbit and the eagle live by their instincts, they go for what they like and avoid what they don't want. They live completely instinctively.

-Well, what if you live instinctively and shut down this complex value and analytical system?

-Then, Doctor, I would have stopped being a human. I often don't go towards what I like because I think I don't have the right. I often do things that I don't like because it's my responsibility.

Well, if I turn off this value system, there would be no right or wrong, and basically, no choice anymore. Instinct would decide, and I act like a 'living machine.' I would become an animal. As you said, something like a rabbit or an eagle.

-Well done, so you have only two ways; Either live like an animal and act instinctively, or like a human being and feel pain and anguish. I want to say that it seems that the more 'human' someone is, the more pain and concern, the more doubt and hesitance, and the more questions they would have. It is a part of the deal.

I want to say that for those who choose instinctively and automatically and live more comfortably than you, their 'inner human' has not yet been born; they're not yet 'awakened.' They are 'potential humans.' I think you should not envy them. You should feel sorry for them that they could be one step ahead of being an animal, but have remained in an animal state.

-But, in many places that describe or write about great people, they introduce 'calmness' as an important characteristic of those people. I think I'm stuck in the middle of the road, I don't have animal peace, nor human peace!

-Of course, but some have different opinion, for example, Rumi says; "The more conscious he is, the more pain he has, the more awakened one is, the paler his face."

Certainly, great humans have different concerns. It is possible that other humans don't worry about the things that potential-humans worry about. So, when potential-humans see Buddhas, they feel the calm and carefree quality, but they don't understand that humans have much bigger concerns and worries that are incomprehensible to them.

-Do you suggest that I should be like that? So, what am I here for?

-I want to say that if you were not a smart person, other people before me would have offered you a framework of thought about the world, our life and duty towards life, and filled your brain with premade ideas. Under that system, you would have known where we came from, where we are going and why we came! You could believe that this framework was complete, accurate, and correct. Then you would become a machine that worked according to the programs running it! Look around you; many people have turned into something like a washing machine or a vacuum cleaner!

It does its job and doesn't worry about the washing machine, and the washing machine doesn't worry about choosing between washing the clothes or the dishes. Many people are living like this. They put their heads down and do what they are told to do, whether this order is given to them by their family, social culture, government, or economy.

As for those who live instinctively; they're just satisfying their hunger and physical needs. Well, you could be one of these potential-humans, you could be a machine and act according to instructions, or you could be an animal and act according to instinct. But unfortunately, or fortunately, you are none of them, you are a human being! If one day you see that you have no worries except for the money to take your children to restaurant, understand that you too have 'transformed.' You've also become a sheep that bends its head, eats grass, mates, grazes, and sleeps. He's not worried about what will happen to the rest of the flock and does not think about where the herd came from and where it's going. He gnaws on the grass and leaves the rest to shepherds and herd dogs, and of course, to wolves and the butchers! A sheep's life is calm and carefree, my friend. But do you want to live like that?

-It's not about wanting, doctor, I 'can't' live like that, it's like I'm like a sheep or like a washing machine according to 'instinct' or I act according to the 'program.' It's like I don't have the right to choose, just like the sheep or the washing machine can't do other things, I also can't be something else. You talk about 'the choice,' but I don't find any choice here. If my human characteristics, my intelligence, or my literacy have made me unable to be deceived by the ideologies, it means that these programs do not fit this device, which means these 'software' are not installed on this system.

Again, it's not my choice; it's still a system that has features and capabilities and has no right to choose apart from what the manufacturer has installed on it. That is, the manufacturing company has designed some systems in such a way that they can be tamed or domesticated like sheep or dogs, and some systems have been designed in such a way that they cannot be domesticated like zebras or wolves. You see, Doctor, I'm not the one who is choosing. If I had chosen these concerns, I could have at least be proud of myself for choosing a higher life, but right now, I've got no reason to be proud. This life was imposed on me!

-If this life is imposed on you, then why don't you commit suicide?

-Because I think, even if I have such a choice, this choice is imposed on me. It's like a prisoner being tortured to such an extent that he should commit suicide to avoid the torture. Actually, the prison guards had killed him! The suicide of a person who is tortured beyond his physical and mental capacity is not a choice. Even if I commit suicide, this scenario is imposed on me, doctor, isn't it?

-...

-Is my time over?

-No, but maybe we should end this session, I need to think more about your words.

Chapter Seven- Norwegian Wood

As we had a day or two off last week, I decided to read some new books. I remembered the book '*1984*' that you talked about in one of our sessions, and I wanted to buy it from you, but I couldn't find your bookstore. You said it was located above the City Theater, but I couldn't find it.

-I wish you had said that to me so I would've brought that book to you, or you had called me, so I would have given you the exact address. The bookstore is not on the main street. It's in the alley and is a bit hard to find. Did you finally find the book?

-Yes, of course, from a bookstore that sold old and second-hand books. By the way, is this book banned?

-What can I say, Doctor? Here, the line between free and prohibited is not clear. No one has officially banned many books, but you cannot find them in the market easily. On the other hand, drugs are officially prohibited, but you can get them anywhere and easily. Anyway, did you read it? Most importantly, did you like it?

-I haven't finished it yet. I think I have read up to 60 pages. At first, I was only looking for 'Oak Tree café,' but then, I liked the topic. I want to talk about the part where the 'party' defines new literature for society, deletes some words, and invents some.

-Yes, I know which part you're referring to. I found it interesting too.

-I remembered the theories of linguists and language psychologists. What I want to say is that the language framework that is taught to us from childhood sets the base for the framework of our thinking, and if we change the language, people's thoughts and feelings will change. Suppose that there's no word equivalent to 'love' in a language, and the only word that exists to express our pleasant feeling towards someone or something is 'like,' which means you have to love someone no matter how much you love them. To express your feelings, just say I like this person. That's all. Suppose there are no words like 'a lot,' 'much,' and the like in this language. Then, if you were born in such a linguistic culture and only spoke this language, do you basically know 'love'? Could you experience it?

-I don't know, maybe yes, maybe not!

-Yes, I mean this part, 'maybe not.'

-Sorry, Doctor, I can't get the point.

-I mean that you look at the world through coloured glasses that are your language. If you change your glasses, maybe the world, your life, and even yourself will change. You just need to look at it in a different way, in the words of Rumi,

'You held a blue glass in front of your eyes,

So, from your point of view, the world seemed blue.'

-You mean I should learn other languages?

-No, you don't necessarily have to learn a new language, you can speak the same Persian language but change your speaking style. I noticed that you talk dramatically. Your language is allegorical, metaphorical, and poetic. Maybe this is the style of speech and, of course, the style of thinking that makes you so sensitive and emotional.

-Can you explain your point in a way that I understand better?

-Yes, I would, but with your participation. For example, you have a lot of concerns about small and big choices in your life. Because you label your choices as 'right' and 'wrong' either according to the task you have or the result they create.

Let's agree not to use the words right and wrong and instead use numbers in a range between one and eight. If you are absolutely sure about the choice you're making, give it the number eight, and if you're not sure, give it the number one and choose a place between one and eight based on the degree of confidence you have in a choice. Okay?

-Go on...

-Well, for example, you're in your bookstore and someone asks you to recommend a book for a gift to his friend. You ask about that person's education and characteristics, and you find out that he is a 22-year-old student of business administration, a person who works hard, studies and is organized. Now, instead of worrying about whether to introduce 'Bread and Wine' to him or the book 'Four weeks to become a millionaire,' just assign a number from one to eight to each of these books.

-Umm. Well, now I'm getting your point. I shall then give 'Bread and Wine' four or five and that millionaire one, two, or maybe... maybe three!

-See! In the previous style of thinking, because instead of a relative view, you used 'either this or that,' these two books seemed to belong to two worlds. Being different, as if you were supposed to choose between 'Good and 'Evil' and you talked so dramatically about the book proposal to your client as if you were going to enter one of the two camps with this proposal. But by scoring, you can see it on an 8-digit scale.

The difference between these two books is between one and three points, that is, between 25 and 37.5 percent. While in your usual way of thinking, it's as if you were dealing with two 100% different spaces, like Shakespeare's 'being' or 'not being'! Don'y you agree?

-I don't know, I'm thinking.

-Yes, very well. As you think, I will continue talking. I will give another example; the same story of your friend in the hospital, a father who didn't have enough money to admit his sick child, and you were all confused by hearing his story.

-Yes.

-Instead of thinking that such an event was good or bad, give it a number between one and eight. The number 'one' belongs to the scene that you don't like at all, and the number 'eight' belongs to the ones that you completely enjoy.

-Yes, it's natural for me to give 'one' to such scenes. I don't like to see such painful scenes at all.

-Well, now I will tell you alternative scenarios, and then you rate it again.

-Yes, please.

-Well, you must have a beautiful scenario in your mind that happens. For example, in Denmark or Finland, all the people are insured, and the public hospitals do not charge any money for admitting patients. When you compare these two scenarios, naturally, one of them brings to mind a white and bright world and the other a black and dark world. And when you see the bleak world, you strongly object to God, to the government, to the medical system, and to the hospital administration so that you want to scream and cry.

-Yes...

-But now I will give you some other scenarios. One of those scenarios is this, there is a child who has an incurable disease. Even if he is in Finland and is accepted for free, he will die! Another scenario, this child does not need hospitalization.

An inexperienced doctor confused his simple disease with an incurable disease and recommended hospitalization. This gentleman does not have money to hospitalize his child, so he returns home, gives his child some pills and painkillers or herbal decoction, and probably he and his wife pray a lot for the sick child. Well, as I said, the child has a simple disease, a viral fever that stops after 3-4 days, the parents are happy as their child recovered without having to bear the expense and trouble of the hospital. In the end, they also find faith in the fact that God loves them very much, and from then on, they look at life optimistically and with gratefulness. Well, now that instead of two scenarios, we have four scenarios, you should rate each of these four scenarios from one to eight.

-For sure. I think I will give 2 to the case where the child dies despite being admitted to the hospital for free because there can be a worse case, and that is when the child is not hospitalized and has no money and dies at the end! Yes, I would give eight, maybe seven, to the situation where the family is insured, and the child is hospitalized for free and will be fine. And to the situation where the child is not hospitalized but has a simple disease and will recover soon, I'll rate it the same seven or eight.

-Great. So, two cases of hospitalization or non-hospitalization of a child, one of which used to be in the white world and the other in the black world, now both will score between seven or eight points, similarly. Because you expanded the observed scene based on many possibilities before and after it to fill your thinking spectrum. Does the fact that someone is asking for free admission for their child still blow you away? You can say, 'A person begged the hospital for his child's hospitalization,' and you can say, 'A person asked for free admission,' these two sentences create two completely different feelings in you.

-Yes, I think I need to think more about how I think.

-Thank you, think, but think 'one to eight.' For example, instead of saying to yourself, I was thinking wrong until now, rate your previous thinking from one to eight...Then how would you rate it?

-Six, maybe five, maybe seven! I should review the alternative scenarios and then grade it!

- Well, now, if I manage to find your bookstore some day and ask you to recommend a book, what book would you recommend to me?

-Err...let me think for a while. Yes, Norwegian Wood.

- Who is the author? Why that one? How would you rate it?

-It's a book by Japanese author Haruki Murakami, revolving around love, loneliness, and death.

-Oh, why on earth you recommend such a book to me?

-I think that, unlike me, you need to feel your emotions a little more, so apart from its score, I recommend this book to you, so you can develop your emotional side as well!

-And why do you want to do that to me?

-Because I got jealous when I was raving about my dramatic feelings, you were cleaning your pipe, testing the sweetness of your coffee, and keeping the time to declare the end of our sessions.

-My goodness. Ok, I'll submit to your punishment and read this book. Maybe I should reconsider my behaviour in the treatment room as well. But meanwhile, please be a little kinder with me.

-Surely, with pleasure!

-Also, you've stayed twenty minutes longer than your time in this session and I talked so much that I didn't get to turn on my pipe!

Chapter Eight- The Fratricide

I thought a lot about what you said in the previous session, doctor.

-Very good, thank you.

-I feel that although it can be said that the theory of one to eight is helpful, it seems that there's something missing, and it does not fit.

-Well, interesting, what's missing?

-Let me begin here. A week ago, I was reading The New Testament when I came across this sentence from Jesus Christ, 'Be either hot or cold, if you are lukewarm, I shall throw you up!'

-Either hot or cold?

-Yes, it's exactly the opposite of your theory, doctor. Jesus Christ says, don't stand in the middle, make your duty clear, either be this way or that way, you know.

What does it mean to be in the middle? It means keeping all your options, which means eating both from the waste and from the manger. I feel that this kind of being is not a deep life; it's a kind of mere convenience. Is this the sole purpose of life? just to have a good time? So I ignore all the love, epics, ideals, battles, zeal, bigotry, bravery, hatred, screams, and.... a hundred thousand deep and painful human experiences and rate the world from one, two, three, four, five, six, seven, eight to finally be able to feel fine. Is this what life is supposed to be?

Also, in our previous session, you said that being human means that we care, so this way of life is contradictory. That if these concerns are not there, wouldn't we become half-humans?

- ...

-You're looking at me badly, doctor!

-No, no, I'm thinking about your words. Please continue.

-I don't know. I guess we were children when we were taught these black and white concepts, as if any choice is as important as choosing between the "good" and the "evil."

Now, you suggest we rate our choices from one to eight and come to the conclusion that a score of seven, and a score of three or four for someone else, means the difference between these two people is not more than 42 to 57%! It's interesting, Doctor. Instead of thinking about how this will make me feel better, think that once accepted at the macro level, if all people think like you said, what kind of world would we have? A world where the difference between good and bad is about 42%? And when there's no clear line between good and evil and, pain, suffering, worry, doubt, torment. What will life be like if people don't have a conscience, a sense of guilt, a sense of responsibility, and etc.?

- Don't you think that most of the violence in history, which probably places them in the black camp of human history, was the result of idealism? You must have read the book *'The Fratricide'* by Nikos Kazantzakis, haven't you?

-Yes, I've read it.

- Very well, each of the two sides of the battle thinks that they are on the right side and their enemy is absolute evil, evil, and evil. But when we view the lives of those who lined up on both sides of the battle scene, we see the same story, with a difference of 20-30% and not more.

The two sides of this battle are so similar that you imagine two brothers standing face to face pointing at each other. As an impartial third party, you cannot determine which side of this campaign belongs to Ahura (good) and which side belongs to Ahriman (evil). Or regarding love, an English writer said, 'Love is an illusion as if a woman is different from other women.' Really, Laila was different from all women that Majnun would spend his whole life on her?

-Doctor, have you seen the movie *'Sex and Philosophy'* by Mohsen Makhmalbaf?

- No, I haven't. Is it a good one?

- Well, I can't say it's an outstanding movie, but I can say it's meaningful. It depicts love; the hero of the film comes to the conclusion that love is a product of romantic conditions, that is, in a special moment, conditions arise that one person becomes important to another person, while a week later, when those conditions are resolved, that same person is no longer special and unique, or at least he doesn't appear to be that special and unique.

Like the rainbow that you see, but an hour later, it's no longer there. The rainbow is an event, it's an incident, just an incident... and from an outside observer's point of view, it's surprising why Majnun fell in love with Laila when there were more beautiful girls in his tribe. But if, instead of being in love with Laila, Majnun scores the girls between one and eight and concludes that Laila does not get more than five, while Farangis gets six and Farahnaz seven, well, of course, he will be fine. He will become the same ordinary man as he was, but if this story is implemented on a large scale, there are no more traces of Hafez's poems or Shams's sonnets. If we erase love and epic from humanity, what kind of civilization and culture will remain?

-Yes, yes, I think we have entered a paradox!

-Paradox?

-Yes, either way, we go this way or that way, we will end up in a dead end. As they say, without love and epic, human life lacks beauty, and on the other hand, much of the darkness of human history are the product of this idealist thinking, which is necessary for the existence of love and epic. It means that both the beauty of human life is owed to idealism and the ugliness of human history. In the words of Hafez, 'My pain is from my lover, and so is my cure.' That reminded me of the movie *'The Receiver'* by Philip Noys and the famous novel by Aldous Huxley and *'Mira'* by Christopher Frank.

-And in such a situation, what should we do?!

-Well, in such a situation, I prefer to make two bitter coffees, fill my cup and sit down together to Tchaikovsky's *'Swan Lake.'* Or perhaps we should listen to Kitaro's *'Caravanserai,'* or maybe some alternative music?

-I agree, again in the words of Hafez, 'Tell a story about dancers and wine and leave the search for the secret of the world, as no one has ever solved this riddle with wisdom.'

-Let me see what music I have here. You should like this; it's a soft music. Did you go to Cafe S-Z?

- S-Z? No doctor, I've never been.

- I got this from there. A week ago, I was sitting there for an hour, and he had put this music on, I liked it a lot, I don't know its name, but luckily its now on my flash drive.

-Do you have time for coffee shops?

- At least 2 to 3 times a week. Sometimes alone, sometimes with one or two people.

-What a beautiful music! It makes me feel good.

- All right, now talk about the good feeling for a while, whatever comes to your mind.

- Yes, yes, by the way, thank you for the coffee.

-You're welcome.

-Yes, a good feeling is like the feeling of friendship and intimacy, like the feeling of belonging and connection, the feeling that we're not strangers, abandoned and lost, the feeling of being in the homeland, the feeling of being in a familiar place.

-Feeling at home?

-Yes, doctor, it seems that sometimes I'm feeling trapped in a nostalgia, as Rumi says, 'Ever since I was parted from the reed-bed, man and woman have moaned in (unison with) my lament.'

It's like I'm a stranger, like someone who fell here from another planet, and even though he looks exactly like the people of this planet, he's not one of them.

- And this music made you feel like you're at home?

- Yes, yes, as if this music reminds me of something related to my planet as described in the book *'The Little Prince'*. Have you read Antoine de Saint-Exupéry ?

- Oh yes, who hasn't? How so?

-Well, talking about the planet, I remembered the little prince who came to earth from another planet. Yes, I was saying, as if this music reminded me of a familiar place.

- And what kind of place is that familiar place?

- There, my planet, where people depend on each other as if their identity has grown, they're close like members of a family. Doctor, I know families with 3-4 brothers, and even though each of them is married and seems to have an independent life at home, in fact, financially and economically, they are so united, for example, the car of one of them belongs to all of them. There's no difference between my interest and your interest. In my planet, it seems like all people are like that. No one withholds anything from another, and no one saves or hoards on stuff.

-Idealism again... this time of the socialist type! Utopia of Plato, Thomas More, and Lenin? And we know how it all ended!

- I know it's not practical, and it's a utopia. But I think being a human means wishing for this utopia and moving towards it.

- Does it mean moving towards a place that does not exist and cannot exist?

-Yes, exactly! Moving to 'Neverland.' Being eager and waiting and assuming that our efforts are not in vain.

-Even if history has showed that it's a futile effort?

-Yes, doctor, that's exactly what it means. It means believing in the unbelievable; that 2 times 2 equals five!

- And does this make you feel better to believe that 2 multiplied by 2 is five instead of four?

-Yes, it does. And this music seems to make me feel better. It tells me that there's still something that shouldn't exist! Have you heard this poem?

"Dry, wired, wooden, dry skin,

Where does this heavenly voice come from?"

In my opinion, the poet is referring to this impossible thing. As a rule, this wire, skin, and dry wood of an instrument should not be able to create such a tender feeling, but they do. It's like dreaming at night; you're in a garden full of fruits and you pick a red apple or a ripe pomegranate from a tree. Then, you wake up and instead of being in that garden, you find yourself in a desert, but just as you are about to despair, you realise that the red apple or pomegranate is still in your hand. How does it make you feel? Unbelievable, but now the garden seems real.

- May I conclude that instead of talking about what life is, it's better to find the sounds that bring joy to your life?

-Agreed. I think you're right; I should follow a special protocol. There must be things or people in my life that 'smell of the homeland,' when that ripe pomegranate is in my hand, I'm not afraid of being in the middle of the desert. I know that somewhere, a fruitful garden is waiting for me; although nothing can be seen except sand and dirt as far as the eye can see, that garden is somewhere nearby, so my hand reached a pomegranate that was on a branch of one of its trees. It doesn't matter if I'm in the middle of an endless desert, at this moment. Whenever I reach out, I can get cold water. I should touch the stream flowing in the middle of that garden and sprinkle handfuls of water on my face.

- Indeed. Adorable! Do you know that our time for this session is over? Recently, I've been too flexible in our schedule.

- It was a beautiful music, thank you.

- And you told me a beautiful story. Thank you. I wish we could find that red apple in our hands once in our life, even when there's no trace of an apple tree nearby.

Chapter Nine- The Farewell Waltz

Doctor, thank you for accepting to meet here instead of your office. This is my hangout, and I preferred our last one here rather than in a therapy session. Do you like the ambience?

- Yes, it has a cozy and warm atmosphere, I should invite you once to SZ cafe... how many different photographs you have on the wall, "Ganadi" next to "Al Pacino" next to "Che Guevara', what does "Charlie Chaplin" photo imply next to Che?

- Nothing really, we just followed our intuition.

- And what will happen if everyone does the same?

- What if they don't? Do you remember our previous session? All roads lead to a dead end. I think I've found the solution, that's why I decided to see you here. I've decided to cease therapy and have a *"Farewell Waltz."* Do you read Milan Kundera? It's an awesome book!

- I agree.

- What would you like to order?

- It doesn't matter, what's your suggestion?

- I recommend a hot coffee with raisin cake, and I'll tell you about the forbidden relationship that I started, a diet based on gut feeling!

- .....?

- You look confused, doctor! I think you didn't approve of the idea that I'm following my heart.

- It's not about approval, your statement is too vague and imprecise! In principle, what desires can be called "gut feeling"? If you want barbecue from the grill, and if you crave sweets from a pastry shop... this is not the call of the heart, this is the effect of the sense of smell on your appetite center! I believe we should have more objective standards, making decisions based on the desire of the heart is like building a house on water, we need stable foundations for life.

- Stable foundations?

- Yes, stable foundations.

- But the earth under our feet, as hard and firm as it seems, is a moving round thing rotating around itself and around the sun in the middle of an ocean of vacuum or antimatter. In addition, it's made of millions of atoms and molecules moving and shaking at a strange speed right now. Despite this, we are sitting firmly on our seats in the oak tree cafe and wouldn't fall from the chair. People used to think that the earth was like a big plate on the horns of a very big cow, which itself was on a giant turtle, which was swimming in the middle of an ocean! The existence of life is almost impossible!
At any moment, the turtle may go deep into the water! And every second the cow may shake its head and that plate will

fall, but with all these possibilities, we're still living. Although nowadays, people no longer accept the cow and turtle theory, our situation is no different from that model in terms of the slim possibility for our existence. We're completely "hanging" in there, spinning and oscillating, but something is holding us, we can call it "gravity" as per physicists, or call it "love" as the mystics say!
Doctor, do you enjoy this music?

- Yes, it's beautiful, did you choose it?

- I thought you should've liked it.

- Thank you, but, I'm still worried about what will happen if everyone follow their heart, won't an "unsafe anarchy" be created? Human nature is selfish and self-centered, if there's no common law, the law of the jungle will rule, violence, rape, etc.

- And is it possible to reach a common commandment, doctor?! Isn't it as impossible as the red apple in our hand when we wake up?! Despite all the laws, instructions, and religions, the human society seems more violent and chaotic than the situation in animal world, doesn't it?

- You see, us humans are among the animals that are interested in group life, that is, if they have to act according to their heart's desire or in other words, instinctively, they have no choice but to live in a group. The basis of social life is based on the acceptance of common rules. For example, assume an intersection, the traffic rules and the presence of traffic lights prevent cars from crashing into each other, but suppose we leave the rules aside and everyone is supposed to do what they want, then what guarantee is there really that you and I, won't have a car crash in the middle of the crossroad, moving at the same time?

- But doctor, such law does not exist on a wide scale, if it did, the entire length of human history was not spent in war, conflict and killing.

- It's true that mankind has not yet reached a universally agreed upon law, but this does not mean that we should replace something called "The law of the heart" for what has not yet been established. Leaving its place empty will make the search continue, but if we put a fake idea in place of it, then we would not notice something important is missing and we would stop our search, as a result, we would remain in the same state of hanging for good.

- How do you know that the lost law is not the following of the heart? Maybe a higher consciousness regulates and manages the hearts and it's enough for everyone to act according to their gut feelings so that everything falls in its right place.

- This theory of yours has already been proposed by another person, but in a different way; "Bernard Mandeville" states something that was finally documented by "Adam Smith", the father of liberal economics. This person believed that everyone should think about their own interests economically and not worry about others, if everyone is look for their own interests, " an invisible hand" would provide collective benefits. Bernard Mandeville's selfish beehive theory and Adam Smith's expression of the invisible hand did not work, that is, when people act selfishly for their own interests, the invisible hand didn't work! Yes, sir, that simple! Instead, discrimination, inequality, corruption, insecurity, poverty, and psychological pressures are increasing day by day. Hoping for an invisible hand is a false hope in my opinion.

- God! I was hoping that I had found a way to feel better. And now you are bringing it to a dead end! Doctor, do you want to make me feel better or worse?

- I don't want to make you feel worse, but I know you're a smart person and even if I don't, you'll wake up in a few days and see that red apple in your hand. It's not you, in my opinion, if you have a stable bad mood, it's better than being happy for a few days and then messing up again. These fluctuations bother you more, I imagine that ups and downs put more pressure on your physical and mental system.

- Do you mean you can't do anything to make me feel better?

- Honestly, no. Do you know why? Because I'm coming to the conclusion that we need a little "stupidity" to be happy, and if someone lacks that little amount of foolishness, they cannot have lasting stable happiness!

- I'm sorry, then what were you doing? I mean, what's the point in psychology?

- I've been thinking about this for several days. I know that not only genius minds like Nietzsche, Dostoyevsky and Schopenhauer were not happy people, but many of the great minds in our specialized field like Freud or Jung were not cheerful, as their biographies and writings show. It's a complicated situation, when people are not in a happy mood, they go to a psychoanalyst to find happiness, while the pioneers in this field were not happy themselves!
Even the definition of a happy person is not so agreed on. Do you know what's the situation like? A driver who has a

passenger in his car who wants to go to a good place, while neither the passenger, nor the driver is sure about the concept of a good place, and whether what's good for him is good for his passenger as well.

It reminds me of the poem, 'I'm drunk and you're crazy, who will take us home?' I know for sure that most of my professional colleagues are not doing better than their clients! They're as confused and helpless as their clients in solving the problems of their lives! It seems like the story of therapy is a game in which the client and the counselor make an agreement so that one comes in a bad mood and then leaves in a good mood, like a role, like a play! In fact, if the counselor and client are both good actors and have a high desire and ability to play the role, psychotherapy will be successful! Unfortunately, it seems that neither you nor I are capable actors, that is, none of us can believe the role we took on.

- Wow, thank you for being so honest.

- Do I have any other choice?

- You could've blamed me for the failure of the therapy and accuse me of resisting recovery and hindering the progress of treatment!

- What benefit would anyone get from that?

- At least you could've loved your job and tell yourself, "I'm doing something important and useful". But how do you want to continue your sessions after this confession?

- I was never a good actor, I couldn't play any roles! I simply couldn't lie, not to myself, not to others. What do I know? Maybe I continue my work while laughing at it, maybe I open a bookstore like you, or a cafe like your friend! Well, the only difference is that I would name it "Freud Cafe".

- Hang on, was this my farewell party with you, or your farewell party with your profession?

- What's the difference? When you reached a dead end, that meant I also reached a dead end. As the poem goes, "The sons of Adam are members of one family."

- Well, these last words of yours, with all their bitterness, somehow made me feel better! Do you remember I said that you feel very lonely when no one understands you? I don't feel alone, at least I'm not alone in this dead-end alley. This calls for a celebration!

- I'm glad. How would you celebrate?

- I'll order two drinks with fresh lemon and salt, and I shall ask my friend to play "Desperado" soundtrack, how does it sound?

- Can't think of a better suggestion, let's do it.

Federal Republic of Puppets

Chapter One-Conflict

I scrape my pipe and remove the burnt tobacco from the mat. Sticking the German filter in a Dutch pipe, and at this moment, the door opens.

-Hello.

-Hello, welcome.

-I'm your colleague, Dr. Niakan.

"Nice to meet you, Doctor." As a sign of respect, I half rise and sink back into my big chair.

-Thanks, actually, I'm a pathologist.

-Please come in. How can I help you?

She pauses anxiously. It's normal. All the seats in this room are 'hotseats.' Confession room, lesson room, punishment room, encouragement room, forget house, etc., all of these are included in the title of 'treatment room.'

-Are you asking questions, or should I start?

-Black chess pieces are mine, so the game starts with you.

-Where should I start?

-It's simple, what brought you here?

-Honestly, I've been contemplating on coming to your office for a long time. I had heard your praise from many people, and I always thought I should visit you one day.

I fill my pipe with Captain Black Royal and press down with my fingers. I ask for permission to light it.

- Yes, cool. I don't smoke, but I like the smell.

I have never heard no in response to my request about the pipe.

There must be a reason why no one has said 'no,' and some hypotheses come to my mind,

1. A naive hypothesis, all people like the smell of a pipe.

2. A sociological hypothesis, Iranian people have not learned to say no to those in power.

3. A psychological hypothesis, I have developed the ability to recognize my clients in the first moment of a session. I take the permission from those who would not object.

My mind searches for the next hypothesis, and at the same time, I light the purple lacquer lighter and smoke the pipe. The thick red and black tobacco smoke swirls around my face. Now I'm in the middle of a halo of light, like religious icons, and I have the possibility to influence her more. Discourse of power! I take a few deep drags as she's still wondering how to begin.

I shake my head with all the puppets in it, which means I'm waiting to hear. The puppets inside my head are falling on each other. Some of them are screaming; some crying; some cursing F words such as Mother...!

They rest stay silent and only their face colour changes and their cheeks blush and turn rosy.

- Honestly, I don't even know what my problem is. I just know that I'm not feeling well, as if somewhere in my body hurts, but I don't know where! It seems that something is wrong, but I cannot locate it. Can't you examine like other doctors or do tests and ultrasounds? Can't you diagnose without my help? I really don't know what my problem is!

-Well, it's okay, we'll drink coffee and chat. Little by little, the puppets in your head start talking, and the puppets in my head tell me what's wrong.

I take the cups, pour two teaspoons in each and fill them up with coffee.

-Sweet or bitter?

-No sugar, thanks. I'm on a diet.

- I don't use sugar. I can offer sweeteners; I'm diabetic.

-Oh, thank you, then please, sweetener.

I fill the cups with boiling water and put the flask of boiling water away. I put her coffee in front of her and stir mine. Now I have to start talking.

-What do you do besides medicine? Your interests, conflicts, and your daily activities?

- Housework with reluctance, a husband with indifference and care and upbringing of children with nervousness.

-And?

- Books, music, travel, my friends. That's it!

- Well, we have gathered some information for this session.

-Really? Was it a lot of information?

- Yes, of course, now I know that you are a woman who dislikes the 'traditional female gender roles.'

- How? Don't you judge too soon?

-No.

I take a sip of my coffee and light my pipe again. She waits and looks impatiently, and I indifferently take two deep puffs on my pipe and blow the thick smoke far away and look at the path of the smoke. One of the puppets says, 'Are you waiting for the oven to heat up and then sticking the bread?'

I answer, 'By sitting on this hot seat, she has given me the consent!' The puppet sticks out its tongue and makes a smiley face. The corner of my nose rises which means 'get lost.'

-No, I'm not quick to judge. When you were talking about house chores, having a husband, and children, you looked like you felt disgusted. The expression on your face was as if you are forcefully eating excessively unpalatable food.

When you mentioned books, music, travel, and my friends, I saw a spark of passion in your eyes, and the tone of your voice became melodical like a song.

- A song?

- Yes, I heard a song in your voice, like the soundtrack of the movie *'No End'* by Krzysztof Kieslowski. A beautiful but sad song.

-Why sad?

-Well, probably. I repeat again, probably, you enjoy these things, but at the same time, you feel guilty; that instead of taking care of the house and family, you read books. For example, the book...

- *'The island'* written by Merle. (French novelist Robert Merle).

- Aha! You walk in the Pacific islands with Tahitians and collect bananas, but at the same time, you know that this is not your home, and you should return as soon as possible. The later you come back, the more work needs to be done, then you have to do all the housework with some impatience and anger, and then...

-I scream at anyone who's in front of me!

-Exactly! Your coffee is getting cold.

She picks up the coffee and stirs. With the spoon and the glass, she goes deep in her thoughts, and before the glass approaches her lips, she lowers her hand,

-Doctor, do I have schizophrenia?

- Schizophrenia? How did you come up with such a strange idea?

- Schizophrenia involves fragmentation of mind, and I think my identity is fragmented, I live in several worlds, and all of them are half!

- No, no, what you're saying in our language means conflict in feelings, values, and beliefs that are incompatible with each other, (They pull this way towards the happy, the other way towards the unpleasant). The ship will either break or pass in the stormy waves.

- My ship is broken, doctor!

- I see, have you seen the movie *'Cast Away'* featuring Tom Hanks?

- Yes, it was broadcasted on TV.

-Yes. Now you're Tom Hanks, and this is the island...

-And what about you?

- I'm the basketball that Tom Hanks drew a face with his own blood on and named it 'Adam'; I'm that kind of man.

She is laughing, and I have time to smoke my black pipe for a while. I wonder if it's a symbol for mysticism in Hafiz poems or following on the footsteps of Freud and Jung.

Chapter Two-Family Size Soda

My hands are cold, I press them in my pockets. The remains of last night's autumn snow are on the ground, I have been sitting in my chair for 6 hours, listening to people's pain, and at the same time, the puppets in my head have been talking, and I am trying to find the most correct answer among all the chatter. I have shortened the long hours with coffee and pipe, but the pressure of time accumulated from human suffering has weighed down on my head, and I am physically tired. I need to calm down the puppets before I go home. I enter the 'Zist' shopping center and go straight to the showcases and jewelry stores, Neyshabour turquoise, Lal agate, ruby, emerald... My eyes are filled with rings and rosaries, and the puppets calm down. In the window of a ring shop, women's wigs are also arranged... 'Augh!'... I feel sick. I don't see any similarity between the wigs and the beauty of rosaries and the turquoise ring.

Another jewelry store posted a paper behind the window, 'Snake bead and dream catcher are available.' The puppets wake up, and one of them says, 'Belief in superstitions and magic! This is what it is!' The other puppet answers, 'By the way, it seems quite modern to me; If things like a snake's bead can create love and affection, it means that love and affection are physicochemical processes, so this is a materialistic view of human beings and human virtues. The puppet's speech reminds me of the movie 'Perfume' and Milan Kundera's books. I feel stubborn that my efforts to put the sounds to sleep have not been successful, and now I should go home with all this noise.

I ring the doorbell. My chubby son, Saleh, answers, 'who is it?' He sees me and opens the door. I call again. Saleh answers, 'What again?' I ask, 'Do you need anything from supermarket?' He pauses and says, 'Soda.' His shy smile is accompanied by shame, he knows that soda is not good for his excess weight, but he likes to eat pasta with soda. Puppets start talking, one of them says, 'Why didn't you say that soda is not good for you?' Are you a father? Maybe the child likes to eat poison, do you have to give it to him?' The frowning man shakes his head with regret, raises the corner of his nose and hates me! Another puppet speaks in support of him; he has taken on a self-righteous and expert look; he doesn't hate me; he is just giving 'ingenious' instructions, 'In Iran, the per capita consumption of dairy products is half of the world, while the per capita consumption of carbonated soft drinks is 4 times the per capita It is average in the world.'

When are we going to be civilized? When are we going to live healthy? Another voice comes to my help, 'Saleh has the right to choose, and the right to choose means the right to make a mistake! If his father tells him today, I won't allow you to drink, tomorrow, the rest of the people in power will give him other dos and don'ts, and he would be used to obeying. The fact that we don't become civilized and live healthily is rooted in the fact that, like buffaloes, we run after the buffalo in front of us, and if it jumps into the abyss, we also jump into the abyss.'

I want to hit my head against the wall. Standing in the crowded supermarket until it is my turn. Black family size soda is freezing in my hands. Someone shouts in my head, 'God! Help me! Tell me what to do?'

Chapter Three- The Pragmatist

70-year-old Mr. Seyed, wearing green gloves and a white beard, is sitting in front of me, asking for help, 'I'm embarrassed in front of my wife.' I understand what he means. He is 70 years old, has high blood pressure and takes two types of medicine. According to Saadi Shirazi, in the sixth chapter of Golestan, his cane is no longer working. One of the little men in my head says, 'Tell him what Osho said; life has seasons, and each season has its own fruits, so eat the fruit of the same season in each season and don't bother yourself with the fruits of another season!' Another voice says, 'What tasks do you assign to people? The old man will be embarrassed in front of his wife. You should help him as a doctor!'

The puppets' conversation continues. I start to write the script when I heard a puppet shouting, 'Damn you! You are a intellectual whore! Instead of showing people the healthy way to live, you take the money and help them in the same way they are going.' I take a deep breath and exhale with a sigh.

He says, 'Doctor's fatigue. May God give you strength and health to help us, poor people.'

I give a forced smile, writing Tadalafil I say in my heart, 'It didn't work for me, God willing it will work for you, Seyed!' And again, a puppet shouts, 'God willing! Again, one of the language rituals, a word that used to mean something once but now has lost its meaning. You live by habits, not by analysing mind. Shame!'

Mr. Seyed shakes hands and leaves, and I call my secretary, 'Will you give me a short break?' I see his smile from behind the phone, 'Sure!'

I go for coffee and a pipe, and at the same time, Mrs. Haydeh starts singing in my head,

'Drunkenness doesn't cure my pain anymore.'

****

The next client is a 16-year-old teenager who is afraid of 'earthquakes' and, as a result, sleeps with his mother and father up to this age. They are humiliated by him.

His uncle came to me from America in summer, and thank God, the treatment went well. The puppet screams, 'Thank God? Linguistic rituals again?'

Now the uncle is sending the nephew to me. Ever since the Bam earthquake, this teenager is afraid of the earthquake. Every sound makes him jump at night. If he doesn't sleep next to his parents, he won't sleep because of the fear of the earthquake.

The man with the turban in my brain moved the robe over his shoulder and said, 'Tell him to recite the prayer (if the earthquakes) at night and blow around him with his mouth, then he will sleep easily!'

The same guy who was sensitive to 'linguistic rituals' lost his control and started cursing. I blocked his mouth; it was ugly and rude. 'Control yourselves. Civilizations talk to each other, you two live in the same head, and you can't learn non-violent discourse?' I said to the puppets.

I realize that the parents of the teenager are still talking, and I don't understand what they are saying. No problem, I'll take care of it. I request the parents to wait in the waiting room so that I can talk to 'Mahdi' alone.

He is a good boy, one year younger than my son Sohail. Like my son, he prefers to study humanities, but his parents are not 'Democratic' like me and tend to manage his life choices, 'How do you know what is good for you? Humanities are being expelled from the country. Sit down and study to become a doctor!' What should I say? They didn't come for a speech about the importance of humanities. They are here so that I could send their child to his own bedroom!

The customer is always right!

I sent him to his bedroom after two sessions with the help of 'Richard Bandler' and 'Goenka' techniques and receive my payments.

'After all, you aren't a prophet to carry the grief of the nation,' Says one of the puppets in my head. He is the pragmatist.

Chapter Four- Richard Bandler

This time, Dr. Niakan talked more readily. As soon as she sat down, I started pouring coffee and while I was lining up the cups, she started talking.

-The most important thing is that I deal with my child badly, and I know it's not the right thing to do. Anyway, I was responsible for him coming to this world, and I'm also responsible for his future. Whether I'm bored, depressed, angry, or as you say, I hate the traditional role of women, he's a child and has no mother except me. If you are going to fix one thing, please help me stop barking at him like a dog and then regret it like a dog!'

One of the puppets in my head starts barking, another pretends to bite, and the third grabs his stomach and laughs. I say angrily, 'Aren't you ashamed? Laughing at my patient? Aren't you ashamed to make fun of a troubled person?'

Her tears flowing, take me out of the world of puppets and I offer her tissues. She thanks and carefully wipes the tears from her eyes so as not to ruin her eye make-up. My heart is burning for her, and I want to say something but that mean voice is shouting in my head, 'If you could, you would have helped yourself,' and with his words, I immediately remember the times when I went home tired from the office or clinic and Sohail and Saleh were fighting, I did the only thing I could do at that moment, I would shout at both of them.

I sometimes sip on boiling water to wash that burning sensation from the bottom of my throat. And then the puppets, sad and silent, with tears in their eyes, sat in front of me and looked at me. I wanted to shout at them too, but my throat was burning, and my power is exhausted, like the flash of a camera that has discharged its electric capacitor and now cannot light up until it is charged.

Today is one of those days when I am exhausted, and I don't feel like doing anything, but as per preplanned appointments, I had to come to the office. My client has wiped her tears, but despite her efforts, she got black on her cheeks, I waited for one of the puppets to laugh at her, but none of them paid attention to me and my client.

She says, 'You don't want to talk today?'

Well, I can't say, 'No, I don't want to talk, or I don't feel like talking today.' I quickly get myself to the front of the brain system and start to talk.

-Are you comfortable reviewing one of those angry outburst scenes? Exactly one moment before the explosion. A moment before you start barking and biting the kid?

She smiles, and her eyes move upwards and left, and I understand from Mr. Richard Bandler's lessons that she is reviewing scenes from the past, up and left!

She shakes her head which means, 'Good? What next?'

I have started walking with my pipe. 'Now see, that is, feel, exactly where that feeling of anger, explosion or whatever you call it is gathered in your body. In another language, 'where is the physical equivalent of this feeling in your body?'

Her eyes immediately go down and to the left, and I go forward with a victorious smile.

Chapter Five-The Holy Spirit

The seventh treatment session with Mrs. Niakan and we no longer discussed everyday issues but dug her fantasy world. The first layer of his fantasy was 'Spider Woman.' I chose this name for her fantasy. When she said that, I remembered Akira Kurosawa's Redbeard, the girl, the lover of the wealthy man who was locked in a cell at the end of Dr. Redbeard's hospital because it was dangerous for men to be free.

He hunted men like a female spider. He called them to the bed of self-immolation and then, by plunging the rods of her hair back into his victim's throat, would kill them. Ms. Niakan also called many men to love games with this fantasy, smashed their heads against the wall, and enjoyed humiliating male spiders.

We passed through the first layer of fantasy. At a deeper level, she had a fantasy to become a psychiatrist. She liked to sink into a big chair and infiltrate into the secret world of people, just like I did. But beneath this fantasy, 'Spider Woman' was also present.

This time she chose male spiders as clients. We passed this layer as well. Today, in the seventh treatment session, we opened a new layer of her fantasies. She liked to experience 'being a whore.' In this treatment method, I enter the fantasies of my clients and rewrite the scenarios of their fantasies, like in the movie Inception. The director puppet was thinking about what role to enter the 'prostitute' fantasy. In the role of a customer? In the role of an aunt? A second wife? Or like the movie 'Under the Light of the Moon' in the role of a cleric? Will it change her life?

I knew that 'spider woman' was also hidden in the depth of the role of the prostitute. Why was hunting male spiders so appealing to her? Was she ever hunted before? Poi-rot twirled his mustache and looked for a clue. Remember, one of my clients gave me this nickname. He had an accident in Malaysia and died. I tried a lot to help him, but because I tried 'a lot,' I was not successful. I spent a lot of time on him and got too close to him, I could no longer use the discourse of power, and the discourse of knowledge was not powerful enough.

I believed Freud in his treatment scenario. Maybe I could have helped him if I had observed a Freudian therapeutic distance or, in the words of Christian Bobin, a 'sacred distance.' I had acted too Jungian and had undergone a process that Dr. Shariati calls 'the tragic end of Jung's life' in his book '*Humanism and the Selfless Man*'.

I was drowned in these thoughts when the Sherlock Holmes puppet hit my forehead a few times with his long pipe and woke me up, 'Hey Poi-rot, don't fall asleep in the middle of work, take it seriously.' I frowned and said, 'This is a part of the work; my associations are also part of my work. Sigmund Freud said that the therapist should be in a state of free-floating attention.'

My feeling tells me to opt for the Freudian method and maintain my distance with this client. So, I choose the role of a cleric to step into her fantasy.

Chapter Six- Theodora

Bahram complains of loneliness and says he has humiliated and ridiculed others in the past, and no one is willing to be his friend and companion. He is studying French and is in his final year.

He says that his university classmates are forming many friendship groups, but he is not accepted in any. He gives them the rights to feel that way. In the first two years of university, his job was to tease his classmates. According to his words, he is a master of destroying others and enjoys this skill, but now that he is alone, he regrets that behavior. Well, I have no knowledge and skills in the field of friendships. What is relevant to my profession is discovering the root of Bahram's behavior pattern. It is obvious that such behavior can only come from someone with a strong sense of inferiority complex.

As a psychological defense mechanism, such a person takes the upper hand; that is, before others humiliate him, he crushes that person in such a way that others do not have the will to offend him. A man shouts, 'Counterattack before the attack.'

Adler puppet with his big belly and round glasses sits in my chair and explains the inferiority complex, defense mechanisms and inversion to Bahram.

Bahram is smart and he gets it. Now he is also curious to know where this deep feeling of inferiority came from. I dig into Bahram's past, especially his childhood, but I don't get any major achievements. I expect Bahram to have been severely humiliated and ridiculed at some point in his life and to have been hurt without defense, and after that secret burning, that emotional wound has led him to this destructive psychological defense; 'Kill to live!'

But no matter how much I search, I don't find such an incident in his life. Maybe the wound was so deep that he anesthetized himself to avoid pain, 'Active Forgetting,' like the lack of historical memory of the Iranian nation. If this is the case, I will have to spend a lot of time, so much so that he reveals the missing pieces of the puzzle amid his scattered words, and cleverly put them together.

Freud's puppet winks at Adler, which means my method works better here. Adler embraces his indifference and cleans his glasses.

'I'm a Christian Buddhist,' says Bahram, who believes in reincarnation.

'What do you mean?' I ask.

He says, 'I have a Buddhist view of Christianity. For example, I deeply believe in successive lives, reincarnation.'

The Sherlock Holmes puppet jumps in and says, 'Until Freud and Adler have discovered something from Bahram's past that would justify his inferiority complex, enter this game, go looking for past lives like Dr. Brian L. Weiss in the book 'Many Lives, Many professors.'

I have a little doubt, but I'm a pragmatist, so I nod in agreement. A few of the puppets lose their balance and fall, and the one who is belligerent starts swearing. I can't hear myself, but right now, I have more important things to do than to deal with a rude secret puppet.

-Well, let your imagination run free to see an imaginary picture of your previous reincarnations. Maybe the origin of this feeling of inferiority is rooted in your previous lives.

He pauses for a brief moment, but he accepts. It's a pleasant game for him. I ride his beliefs and smile triumphantly, but the critic in my head doesn't let me enjoy this success. He shouts, 'Does the end justify the means?'

I try to ignore him, but he jumps in front of me and shouts, 'Death to Stalin!' I try to keep my calm, 'Look, my brother, people come to me to reduce their bitterness, not to hear the truth. This is our contract. I act according to the contract. This is what they call professional ethics, ethics according to Sir David William Ross...'

He interrupts me, 'Hey boy, we'll get to you too, scoundrel intellectual!' I know he is referring to Dariush Mehrjoui's book *The Grand Inspector and the Rogue Intellectuals.*' I want to defend myself, but he doesn't allow me to speak, 'Hey dear sir, you know well that fascism is based on rogue intellectuals, and you, you are a scoundrel intellectual. Ethics? Have you forgotten that Karl Marx considers professionalism as the spell of a capitalist society, Mr. Ernesto Che Guevara?'

This kind of sarcasm drives me crazy. I know the voice is not giving up, but I am also determined not to lose the golden opportunity to treat Bahram. 'You're caught in Scientism, bro!' I shout. In the words of Robert Merle, 'We have to act until the end.'

He grins, 'Action! Guerrilla culture! Guerrilla without morals." I want to punch the puppet but right then Bahram speaks and pulls me out of the fruitless conversation with the puppet.

- Yes, I found my previous reincarnation. I lived between 1850 and 1900. In France, I was a composer and a piano teacher, an outstanding, well-known, and influential composer... I think I was a woman. At that time, few women had reached such a degree in art and philosophy.

I take a deep breath; the game is going well, so I continue. The puppet makes rude movements and leaves. He knows that at this stage, I will not give up the game. I continue, 'What was your name?'

-Theodora... Theodora Austin.

-Well, in that reincarnation of yours, I was also present as a priest, the priest who came to your deathbed to comfort your soul.

And you confess to your pastor. You admit why you die with a bag of inferiority complex, feeling the humiliation you have brought to this life.

-Honestly... I committed suicide. I committed suicide because I felt humiliated. I remember I did something I was ashamed of, and the only way to escape that scandal was suicide.

-That's why you transferred the karma of that life to this life. You ran away from the problem instead of facing it. The things we run from follow us, even from one life to another.

-Does that mean that even if I commit suicide in this life, I will not get rid of it?

-Not at all! This is the worst approach because your next life will be spent on this.

The critical puppet passes in front of me, smiles, and mutters under his breath, 'fraud,' and he leaves.

Chapter Seven- The Oedipus

Farshid and Marzieh visit me for premarital counseling. Both have been my students and colleagues. Farshid studied psychology and Marzia is a doctor. They met each other at parties of mutual friends and have been in a relationship for some time now. I know both almost very well. When they were my students, each of them came to me for separate counseling sessions. I would hear the life story of each of them for an hour and guide them accordingly. Both had a divorce in their previous marriage. Marzieh experienced a divorce that was full of stress and conflict because she had cheated on her husband. On the other hand, Farshid had entered into a romantic relationship with another woman to take revenge on his wife, who had betrayed him. His story also ended in divorce after a tense period.

During several months of the relationship, Farshid and Marzieh had undergone a rough phase that was full of uncertainty, stress, and anxious thoughts. Marzieh had disappeared for a day and later admitted that she fancied a man in the car wash, they exchanged phone numbers and had a date the same day, which led to sexual intercourse afterward. Marzieh suffers from cyclical mood (cyclothymia), mood swings, she takes drugs and one during impulsive ups and downs has sex with masculine men.

Now, these two people have decided to get married. They both have studied psychology and know the consequences of this marriage. With all the various emotional and sexual relationships that he has experienced, Farshid still lives in the historical era of the myth of virginity, and he dreams that, like in old romantic movies, where a hero saves a woman from prostitution by his immense love, he could change Marzia's and remove her impulsive sexual relationships and make her a dedicated housewife just like his mother.

I ask Farshid, 'You know that Marzieh is not the virgin of your nostalgic dreams?'

He replies, 'I know. She told me that she has slept around with a thousand men!'

I say, 'Okay?'

-They were not enough for her, each of them lacked in one area, but I am the one. I know both the art of communication and the art of sex!'

I smile at Farshid's inflated self-confidence, he understands what it means and says, 'Okay, increase her medication, if her mood is stabilized, she won't get into impulsive relationships.'

I reply, 'she has stopped her medication many times, she will stop taking it again. This pattern has been going on for years.'

They came back after a few weeks. They had decided to get married, and they came to inform me with an invitation card. I stayed silent, thinking of it as a classic example of neurosis. Self-awareness has not led to salvation, just as Oedipus' precognition did not save him from the spell of the Gods. I ask, 'If your relationship is good as is, why do you insist on registering it in a marriage? And if your relationship is not good, why do you insist on continuing it?'

Farshid, who insists on getting married more than Marzieh, answers, 'In both of our birth certificates, divorce is recorded once, it will not cause a problem if happens again.'

I ask, 'What's the advantage of registering your love in your birth certificates?'

He says, 'We won't have a problem going to the hotel anymore; we have a marriage certificate.'

A few months ago, they had traveled to Shiraz to experience the romantic May with the fragrance of spring flowers. Although they had reserved two separate rooms in a five-star hotel, when they went to a room at the end of the night, the security guard of the hotel was like a pinpoint missile. The morality police had spotted them, and until dawn, the love pigeons were held in custody, and at the time of the morning call to prayer, they were released after being fined.

('In Iran, a man and a woman do not have the right to be together or travel together and stay in the same room without having a marriage certificate! It is illegal!' Translator)

I think to myself, 'Psychophobia and totalitarianism are perfect complements to each other.' Freud's puppet picks up a cigarette, Che Guevara's puppet gives him a lighter!

***

Nine months later, Farshid and Marzieh got divorced. Freud used to say, 'Psychoanalysts are secular priests!' Now Farshid is sitting in front of me as he is mourning. The Oedipus, looking for his mother's gaze in Marzieh's eyes and Hollywood stars in her body, is now looking for Antigone by his side.

Chapter Eight- Christian Bobin

It was decided that Dr. Niakan would turn her fantasy into a story and give me a role in her stories on her own initiative. My way of channeling his fantasy didn't work. I encouraged her to express her fantasies freely. Her first writings were clichés and repetitive. A mish mash of the novels that she had read. I encouraged her to read surreal works and then start writing. I introduced her a few examples of surrealism novels, which I enjoyed a lot, *'Murshid and Margarita'* by Mikhail Bulgakov and *'Session in Aleppo'* by Jaafar Modarres Sadeghi.

In the next session, she records her panic attacks in her writings and establishes a surreal dialogue with her anxiety. Our work is going well; we are both satisfied. I guide her novel in such a way that it becomes post-modern, and when finished, I encourage her to create a blog and put her novel in it. Great results. She gets approval from her readers, and the artist inside her wakes up.

In the next session, she goes to her therapeutic relationship and this time she gives me a prominent role in her novel, the same role she wants me to have in the real world, and I manage to establish active transference. Franz Alexander's puppet is sitting on the big sofa in the treatment room, crossing his legs and scratching his head. He seems satisfied.

*****

Contrary to the advertisements of the therapist who referred her to me, I do not find any complex mystery or deep secret in her. I am writing my treatment report for a colleague, thinking to myself, why is this client so interesting to my colleague and not to me? I suppose it depends on the realm of our curiosity, but as I sip my coffee, another idea comes to mind; *The Sacred Distance*.

Christian Bobin, a French writer, said, 'If you look at anyone from a sacred distance, they are a masterpiece, a wonderful work of art, a glorious mystery. If someone is not interesting to you; either you are too close or not close enough to them.'

As simple as that.

Chapter Nine-A Father's Signature

I hypnotize Mr. Engineer and take him to his inner house. It is quiet and cold, and he is afraid of the vermin inside the house. The walls are made of cement. I say, look on the cement walls and see what is carved on them. He gazes at the wall but doesn't find it. I tell him to look more, he looks again and finally finds it; it is his father's signature. This short hypnotic journey reveals the scenario of his life to me.

He lives to get his father's approval and he needs his father's signature.

Now I know that to better understand his story, I have to know his father's story, so I write some incomplete sentences for him to complete them,

My father...

My father...

I wish my father,

He ponders and carefully fills in the sentences.

My father is kind.

My father is hardworking and compassionate.

I wish my father was not an orphan.

And I continue the game,

My father is kind, but

My father is hardworking and compassionate.

I wish my father was not an orphan, and in this case,

He carefully completes again,

My father is kind, but he has to show his love.

My father is hardworking and caring but somewhat self-righteous.

I wish my father was not an orphan because he would be calmer and more balanced.

Now I continue the game like this; I put his name instead of his father and rewrite it,

I'm kind, but I have to show it.

I am hardworking and caring but somewhat independent.

And if I didn't grow up with a father who experienced orphanhood, I would be calmer and more balanced.

I ask him to keep these three sentences in front of his eyes the coming week. Our treatment session ends.

*****

I often tell my students that we will never know definitively which client has improved and which is pretending that to please us. And we will never know which one of our clients would not improve or plays the role of 'I will not improve' to spite us. I wish we could have measured our clients' recovery with radiography or a blood test like other doctors. Then, we could have assessed our techniques better. In the current situation, we just walk like the blind and drag the other one behind us in the same darkness, I'm drunk and you're crazy; who will lead us home?

Chapter Ten - Socrates

A woman has come for counseling about her marriage. Her psychologist has also come with her and wants to know my opinion. This lady lives with a man who limits her, threatens, and humiliates her. However, she continues her married life in the hope of changing her husband. She told me that her husband, has stolen the title deed of his old aunt's house and sold her house by forging the documents through bribes and connections he had. Her husband works in a company as a legal expert, but he steals the information and sells it to the competitors.

However, this lady hopes that her husband will change for better to improve their married life. Her husband refused to see a psychologist. My advice to this lady is that she should separate from her husband within one year at the latest and I want the psychologist to prepare her for her independent journey by then.

The fear of loneliness and negative social view on divorced women makes her stay in the toxic marriage. In response to the hope of change, I say to this lady, 'This hope of yours is like hoping that your cherry tree will bear pears next year! This is not hope; it's wishful thinking!'

She leaves the session and I stay with her psychologist. He asked me how recommended a divorce with just one session. I said, 'Some behaviors can be judged decisively, for a man who steals from his aunt and betrays the organization; there's no hope.'

Now the psychologist is gone, and I am left alone with a pen and paper. I ask myself if my judgment was not wrong. The puppet of Socrates comes forward and questions me,

- How do you know that this woman gave you the right information? How do you know that her husband is unchangeable?

And then he shows me a movie about my life and shows me my deep changes. I will resist the Socrates and I am not going to budge. I have indeed changed a lot, but not many things have changed in me. I think life has two aspects: a recurring aspect and an exceptional one. Every rule is full of exceptions. We say that water freezes at 0 degrees and boils at 100 degrees, but this rule only applies when the water is pure and the air pressure is at the level of the open seas, so the water in our house does not boil at 100 degrees. According to Jung, 'Each person is an exception to the rule.' But this exception does not prevent us from ignoring the rule.

Socrates is still busy with challenging questions, but I think that if Socrates was going to make an executive decision for life, he would have to assume non-obvious assumptions as self-evident. Didn't he submit to the verdict of an unfair court? The Socrates puppet is disappointed in me and is now talking to Phaedoris about language, 'Language is both pain and painkiller, creating both understanding and misunderstanding.'

Ludwig Wittgenstein joins them and asks Socrates, 'Do you think the tree has an external existence?'

Socrates looks at him.

Wittgenstein continues, 'No, there isn't. The tree is a game of language!'

I think that skepticism leads to madness, just like certainty. The difference is only in the type of madness!

Chapter Eleven-Departure

Some of the puppets are packing their bags.
-Where to?
-Other places, other lands, other people, other heads!
-Your place in my mind will be empty, I will miss you!
-It won't remain empty, you won't have time to get bored, new puppets are coming.
-From where?
-Other lands, other people's heads!

Nightmares of a postmodern Shaman

Chapter One-The Sacred Throne

The smoke rises from the logs as we move.
The direction of the wind changes every ten to fifteen minutes, and we should change places so that the smoke does not hurt our throats and eyes.

-One is afraid while sitting in front of a psychoanalyst. She thinks that you can see her in her head, of course, I have nothing to hide. Everything in my life is out there, but I don't know why I still feel anxious if someone sitting in front of me could read my mind. It's like your eyes are the predators, tearing apart a person's body to go beyond and see the soul of a person.

As I said, I've nothing to hide, so there's no reason to be afraid of exposing my soul. Maybe I'm afraid that you might misinterpret my intentions. To be honest, I don't believe in psychoanalysis at all. I always tell my friend that it's impossible for someone who knows nothing about a person except a bunch of 'useless and absurd' theories about an unknown thing called the psyche, to figure us out. How can someone decode a person by listening to them narrate their experiences of several decades in only a few hours? Not only that, how can he put a label on the storyteller's forehead that reads, for example, 'Mother's complex.' Well, so what?

At that moment, Mr. Mohammad brings tea and she stops talking. Mohammad offers me sweets but I don't take any. He insists, 'This is different from other sweets.' The amount of insistence is enough to break my diet and put the candy in my mouth, which by the way, tastes like all other sweets in the world.

Maryam wants to continue, but I start talking, 'Let me put your mind at ease. It's true that I'm a psychiatrist, and it's true that I've been teaching psychoanalysis for years, but first of all, my look is not predatory. I don't have a third eye or the eyes of purgatory or the intuitions that some people have or that they claim to have, or that people think that they have. Honestly, I see less in other people than any ordinary person. Every once in a while, there's a person who I thought I knew a lot but turns out I didn't know them at all!

Secondly, and most importantly, I came here for a party, so I'm not going to psychoanalyze you here. Thirdly, which might sound the most interesting to you, is that I have basically given up the work of therapy and just teach and write, so even if you insist, I wouldn't analyze you with the glasses of psychoanalysis. I shall suggest that you give up on me, and instead, I'll introduce a few of my good friends and colleagues to book an appointment with them.'

-Wow! But why?

-What why?

-Why did you stop being a therapist?

-Being a therapist, aside from having the knowledge and skills, requires something else that may not be acquired. For example, the therapist must have a kind of 'therapist personality,' a certain type of personality that differentiates him from the rest, like an artist, who must have a certain type of personality. An artistic personality cannot be obtained by going to a painting or music class, also, a therapist must also have a personality that is certainly not achieved by attending university and taking courses and even by being psychoanalyzed. I don't know how much of this is influenced by genes or archetypes and how much by family, school, culture, and time, but I know for sure that it's not something that can be obtained in the form of a contract with a few years of study.

Anyway, I think that I don't have a therapist personality, so I prefer to teach the knowledge and skills of a therapist. I will teach people who are interested in knowing or would like to do this, and some percentage of them may have that therapeutic personality innately, and those are the people who, in my opinion, can become good therapists in the future. So, rest assured that you're not psychoanalyzed by me.

The direction of the wind has changed again, and we get up again and look for a 'sacred distance,' where we can have the warmth of the fire, without the smoke irritating our eyes. It is not an easy task. We move the chairs several times because while we have to be in the right position towards the fire, we also have to maintain our circle so that we can face each other. This way, we are more likely to understand each other. Finally, each of us finds a temporary place, and we sit in the chairs. This is an opportunity for Fereydoun to take the lead in the conversation.

- Doc, I think you're being unfair to yourself. I'm sure if one day Maryam decides to go to therapy, you're the best option. I'm not a flatterer; I don't give compliments, either. I was in the class of many professors; I'm not a bad connoisseur because I've a lot of experience with different people. I've been between all the professors I met so far and their master classes and workshops. To be honest, I only approve of you and Dr. Gorgani, of course, maybe in a way. Call it arrogance or self-conceit that I'm evaluating my professors, but this is my feeling, and I think that if a therapist requires a special character apart from knowledge and skill, you have that character.

I want to answer, but Maryam jumps in the middle of the discussion, 'Maybe there's another reason why you abandoned therapy and are somehow justifying it to yourself and others.'

'Well, maybe!' I replied, reflecting on her words.

-Probably a 'big gaffe' somewhere, and this blunder made you lose your self-confidence. And because you have a all or nothing personality, now you don't trust yourself at all. You think you don't have the ability to know people, you think you're not qualified as a therapist. You don't have it, maybe you do, but you're punishing yourself for that big mistake.

Maryam is psychoanalyzing me. God! How strange these people are, until a few minutes ago she was saying that she does not believe in psychoanalysis. But now she has become my psychoanalyst. She is analyzing me without my consent and the first label that was stuck on my forehead was 'blunder!' Ironically, she is using the same 'useless and absurd' theories that she didn't accept a few minutes ago. She is commenting on my self-confidence, my personality, and self-punishment like an adept therapist. I think that sitting in the therapist's chair is a special pleasure. It is a pleasure that therapists are addicted to and non-therapists long for. They may start treatment for any reason, different reasons, but then, at least one of the reasons for continuing treatment is that they want to get closer to that sacred and tempting chair.

A chair that centuries ago, the 'shamans' or the witch of the tribe used to sit on, and now a man with a suit, glasses, a goatee beard and preferably with a pipe in his hand sits on it. In my mind, I ponder the temptations to approach the witch of the tribe, magic, miracles, omens, the future telling, fate, power, oh my God!

Magic reinforce the discourse that the world has another layer. Life has a depth other than the everyday, and that means we are not here by a mere accident, and we do not vanish after death. Four existential dead-ends are spinning rapidly in my head, death, meaninglessness, loneliness, and freedom. And the refuge comes in belief in immortality, ideal, love, and principles.

Maryam, happy to sit on the shaman's throne, is staring at me with a triumphant smile, ready to defend the dignity of the analysis she has just presented. Maryam is apologizing for her psychoanalysis and explaining why she said what she said. 'Excuse me, I'm getting too emotional, jumping to conclusions, I don't know anything about psychology. In fact, I've never even read a psychology book in my life. I always hated it. Fereydoun knows that I'm quite erratic and speak up everything in my mind, saying it out loud.'

Now she is explaining about herself, but I am looking at the story in a different way and telling myself that apart from Maryam's temptation to become a shaman and the charm of analyzing others, maybe this 'sense' of Maryam is a third eye. I also wouldn't mind finding a 'guru' who has a third eye and pulls the curtain. I also need miracles, magic, meaning, and transcendence. At the same time, I'm looking into my life to find that big blunder.

****

We are riding towards the city on the highway. It's almost midnight, the breeze is cold. We talked for seven or eight hours non-stop, around the fire before sunset, and after sunset, we curled up around the small electric heater in Fereydoun's villa. Even though the heater of Fereydoun's car is on, it seems as if the ice in my bones hasn't melted yet. My bones are literally shivering. Now Maryam insists that I accept her treatment as an exception, although she still does not believe in psychology, but she thinks that she must talk to me to solve a 'specific' problem. According to her, she must talk to me urgently, so we can comprehend why I left being a therapist.

I don't say 'no' firmly, maybe because I'm not that strong-minded of a person and my boundaries can be messed up by 'insisting.' It could be very well because of my attraction to the cinema – silver curtain, red carpet, camera flash. Maryam is a famous actress, not one of those beautiful actresses that everyone wants to sleep with but one of those mysteries that everyone loves to unravel. Now I'm in the game. My curiosity or rather nosy nature is triggered to discover what secret there is in the life of this beautiful actress that she wants to share with me, maybe she was able to tickle my narcissism as well; someone who doesn't accept anyone is asking me to accept her, desperately.

Chapter Two - The Shaman

The smoke rises from the logs and a cold and strong wind blows. The sound of the river is so loud that we can barely hear each other's voices, but we are not supposed to talk to each other. The shaman's assistant plays the tambourine, without having any specific music or rhythm, he just beats the tambourine every few minutes. The shaman also shakes the big bell in his hand once in a while. It's like a camel bell, neither the beats of the tambourine nor the sound of the bell has any order, but their mixing with the sound of the river creates a kind of symphony of anarchy that keeps me from a slumber.

I drag my chair to the fire so that I don't freeze from the whipping wind. I cover my face with my hand so that the smoke doesn't enter my throat and eyes. After a few minutes, the shaman gets up and sits in front of the three of us, staring right into our eyes, one by one. His assistant continues to beat the tambourine. The third time he sits staring into my eyes, my eyelids become heavy. It feels like some odd force is trying to shut them close. I still hear the roar of the river and the beats of the tambourine, but slowly the sounds around me are changing. Suddenly, the sound of the river is replaced by the sound of torrential rain, and instead of the beats of the tambourine, I hear rowing.

I instantly open my eyes. I'm sitting in an old wooden boat and a girl with almond eyes, wrapped in a clear raincoat resembling a big plastic bag is rowing. I have an umbrella in my hand, but the rain is so intense that my clothes are completely soaked. I look around to register the surroundings around me. We have moved away from the shore of the lake. I can spot a wooden pier and a cottage at the end of the pier, and we are moving towards the middle of the lake. As we move a little further, tiny wooden huts float on the surface of the lake. Each of the huts has a different colour.

I've seen this before in a movie. *'The Isle,'* by Kim Ki-duk. The shaman was right, I am thrown into one of my fantasies, I close my eyes tightly, hoping to return to where I was, but it is impossible. Even when I close my eyes, all I can hear is the sound of the torrential rain and the strokes of the oars on the lake. I open and close my eyes several times, but all in vain. As he said, I'm thrown here and will be stuck here for a year or even ten years. I asked him, 'well, if I stay here for ten years, will my body stay there, by the river, in the middle of the forest? Will you take care of me? Will you transfer my body to another place? Will you feed me with a tube?' He replied, 'No, it doesn't take more than a few minutes or most probably a few hours here, but where you are now, there it takes months or even years. The speed of time passing in these two worlds is different, time is heavy and slow there, compared to here. Where you go, you get the same feeling that you have here because of the passage of time, but every minute that passes here lasts for days or even weeks, and you stay there until the story ends. When I recall his words, I get scared, thinking I might be stuck in this strange land for years.

As I ponder over these thoughts, I panic. I scream and gesture to the boat girl to take me to the beach. She looks at me blankly and indifferently with no reaction and continues rowing at the same pace. It seems that she is used to such behaviours, or that she is in another world and neither sees me nor hears my voice. The umbrella falls from my hand, and the heavy rain pours on my head and face. I let it rain on me. Maybe I'll wake up, maybe I'll go back to where I was. I'm afraid of being stuck somewhere without a way back for years, but I am stuck in this peculiar world as if this is the only reality that exists and my previous life was a dream that I cannot return to.

When you wake up, you cannot go back to a dream, even when you are in a dream, the dream you see is not under your control. You may see the same dream two nights in a row and years may pass but the dream does not repeat even once. And all my previous life, my friends, family, work, hobbies, pains, and joys, have morphed into a dream now, I can't go back to, no matter how hard I try. It is terrifying even to imagine such a thing.

What are they doing now? What happens if I can never go back? Will my body start to rot there? If I stop breathing and my heart ceases beating, once they find my body next to the ashes of a dead stove by a river, will they take it to the forensics to determine the cause of death?

What will my family do next? My children? What will happen to them after me? I'm so scared that I want to throw myself in the lake for a moment, but I am afraid of drowning as always. As much as I want to jump into the lake, the torturous thoughts of being swept away by a tide hold me from jumping. Although this world is a fantasy, I'm still afraid of drowning in water. I don't know if I die here, will I come out of trance there or will I die there too? I haven't asked the shaman before entering this world. I didn't think it was real. I thought it was like an imaginary journey where I could open my eyes whenever I want. I could get up, shake my clothes, splash water on my face, and return to my actual world and life.

But now, it doesn't seem like I possess the will to come out of the trance. I'm stuck in this fantasy, which has turned the trance into a nightmare. No matter what I do, the boater girl is unconcerned. She paddles the boat at the same pace until we reach one of those floating huts. She wraps the rope from the boat around the pole, jumps to the platform, and puts the basket from the boat on the platform. I have no choice. I can't stay under this rain, and I don't have the courage to throw myself in the lake. I take her hand and get up. She opens the sliding door of the hut and enters. I follow her inside. The wooden floor gets wet from the water dripping from our clothes. She doesn't take off her raincoat, but she points me to hang my wet jacket on the hanger installed up the window.

There is a small oil stove in the middle of the hut. The girl lights a match, and the wick of the oil lamp puts on a yellow flame. She plays with the knob, the wick goes up and down and finally, the flame turns blue. She takes the kettle, opens a hatch in the bottom of the hut, fills the kettle with water, closes the hatch, and places the kettle on the stove. She takes out some plastic bags from the basket, containing tea, sugar, bread, and apple with a glass and a spoon.

She gets up to leave. I ask helplessly, 'Are you leaving? What am I going to do here?' She pauses briefly but does not turn to me. It is now clear that she is not deaf, but obvious that she does not understand my language, so she moves further and abandons me. I know this place. In the movie, I have seen that when the rain stops, it's a beautiful place, but not for someone who is stuck here and has left his entire forty-six-year-old life somewhere else. The girl gets on the boat and unties the rope from the pole on the floating wooden isle. She takes her oars and starts rowing.

'Don't go, I'm scared!' I yell desperately. Again, she pauses for a moment but does not turn her face, she paddles and drifts away. I look at her hopelessly, then I close the sliding door and gaze around the hut. The water is still dripping from my jacket, making a small pond on the wooden floor.

I can see the lake through the wooden beams on the floor. In the middle of the hut, a kettle whistles softly on an oil lamp. In one corner, there are two thin blankets for sleeping, and a wooden hatch on the floor that can be raised, then the lake would receive the waste.

I feel my entire life constricted into this one dream, where I'm alone in the middle of a hut roughly the size of a bed or maybe a little bigger. There is no human in sight, no books, mobile, internet, TV, no way out. Stretching out the blanket, I sat on it. I can't give up but also can't fight. I'm confused and terrified. The kettle boils. My only option right now is whether to have some tea or not, that's all. I pull a tea bag out of the box and put it in the metal cup with a handle. Then, I fill it with boiling water and wait for the colour to seep into the boiling water.

Chapter Three-The Safety Net

Maryam and Fereydoun are coming to my house tomorrow. Fereydoun studies psychology and likes to attend Maryam's psychotherapy sessions to learn the art of the work. Maryam had no problem with his presence. On the same day, we set an appointment, and Fereydoun was also scheduled to be there.

'Maryam, you might want to say stuff that you aren't comfortable in my presence,' Fereydoun offered.

Maryam answered, 'You know about all my life, Fereydoun.'

Honestly, I am also more comfortable with his presence. Maybe, as Maryam says, I have made a big mistake and don't trust myself anymore. The presence of an assistant or even an observer will ensure that I make fewer mistakes.

I wanted to see if I have any intuition left. That's why I decided to sit alone with myself the day before the therapy session to see if I can imagine what help Maryam will ask me for tomorrow. I thought to myself if the therapist has something like 'third eyes.' Also, if one doesn't have intuition, what tool is he supposed to use to see the depth of people? An analytical mind? If the analytical mind is given the wrong data, it will analyze it wrongly.

By observing body language? Well, that's one word, people lie more easily with their tongue than with their body language, but people don't always lie consciously. Sometimes they have wrong beliefs, that is, they have already believed in a lie themselves. In this case, the difference between 'evidence' and 'swearing against the evidence' will not be obvious. At the time when people believed that the sun revolves around the earth, their body language must have testified to it while talking about it.

Therefore, the skill of reading body language cannot be a strong thread to hang onto during therapy. Perhaps intuition does not have a spiritual and supernatural meaning, but it is just another name for experience, a kind of analogy, you can say. You get so much into people's behind-the-scenes life that you gradually get a series of 'general patterns' of people's behaviour and relationships. Then you put the data you get from the references in that 'coordinate device,' like solving equations with two unknowns.

In other words, the inexperienced therapist (who has not yet grasped the general patterns) will make a lot of mistakes, until the number of such errors gradually decreases as his hair turns grey. This also means that for years he has made the wrong diagnosis and prescribed ineffective medicine. If this is the case, then anyone who is looking for a psychotherapist should look for someone who has spent years of trial and error to achieve 'reliability' and solid experience and expertise.

If all the people visit an experienced therapist, then on whom should the inexperienced do trial and error to achieve reliability and empirical intuition?

Well, we have a dilemma.

Chapter Four - The Purgatory

I wake up. Seeing the roof of a floating hut above me, I immediately remember where I am. I have never been under such a roof in my previous life. There is no sound of rain. I remember the words of the shaman, 'You are thrown into one of your fantasies, a place where you have imagined living there before, but you have never been there. You might get stuck in that imagination. Maybe for a year, maybe for ten years you will stay there. You stay until the story ends.'

I am scared again. I sit down, contemplating the things that I did yesterday. My impatience had no effect on the course of events, no matter how hard I beat myself against the doors and walls, I would not wake up from this dream. This dream is now the only available reality of my life. I suddenly recall the dreams I had last night. Maybe my dreams could provide a key to my life and the way back to it. I think hard, but I can't remember anything. I push myself again. Maybe this time I could remember something from my dream last night, but I recall absolutely nothing. I stand up, open the sliding door, and step out.

Outside, a thick fog covers the surface of the lake. The air around me is soft, loaded with the fragrances of grass and wood. The high-pitched sound of frogs echoes in the air.

The fog is too thick to make out the shore of the lake, the pier, and the boat girl's cottage. I can only see the blurry shadows of one or two huts nearby. Honestly, this place is beautiful, it's wonderful, but it's somehow quiet, even with the buzzing of amphibians. Maybe when I saw Kim Ki-duk's movie, I wished to spend a few days here – a wish not impossible but improbable. Now I have my dream granted, but I am locked inside it, alone, without a clear way to freedom.

I am worried about my life in the real world. The shaman had said that 'here' minutes or at most hours pass, while 'there' seems like months or years. So, everything was now 'over there' (formerly here) and I didn't have to worry about it. So far, the shaman's words were true, so basically his other words must be true as well. I repeat to myself again, 'Everything remains almost still there because, for every year that passes here, an hour passes in real life.' After last night and until now, 10 to 12 hours have passed, which is not more than a few minutes there. In the eyes of those who are outside the shamanic ceremony, we are a few people sitting around the fire and I have closed my eyes and I am in a trance. According to them, nothing out of the ordinary is happening, and I am sitting in the same position with my eyes closed.

The shaman also shakes the bell on the camel's neck from time to time and his assistant is busy playing the tambourine. Ok, so everything is back to normal there, nothing happened to worry about. Maybe if a painful stimulus hurts my body there, for example, a snake bites my ankle, I will come out of the trance. Like jumping out of sleep, I will jump out of ecstasy and see that I am in my place and take a deep breath and everything will be over, that's it. I feel like I'm dreaming, but I know if I'm dreaming. Why does this story scare me so much? Of course, this internal conversation should calm me down, but it doesn't. Maybe my fear comes from the fact that I have no control over anything here.

Being stuck on a small island in the middle of a lake, I don't know how to swim and don't have a boat, either. All I have is a small breakfast left for me by the girl. I go to the oil stove, light a match and put the stove on. I adjust the wick, boil the kettle, and put it on the stove, then I look in the plastic bag, which contains tea bags, sugar, bread, and apples.

I remember something. Where is my medicine? In the real world, every morning, I measured my sugar, took medicine, and injected insulin. But there is no medication, no glucometer, no insulin, and a syringe in the plastic that the girl has left for me. Well, it makes sense. Since this floating hut is an imagination, and my main body is not here, the food I will eat here will not affect my body there. Hence, I can eat whatever I want without the need to take insulin. Here, this 'ethereal Body' of mine does not have diabetes.

I sweeten my tea with sugar, sit in front of the hut, eat bread, and drink my tea. I try to enjoy myself while I'm here alone, away from the chaotic world. Sweet hot tea, stale bread, a calm lake, morning fog, solitude – everything seems great. The best part of all is this ethereal healthy body, which doesn't need a glucometer, insulin, pills, or food restrictions. However, I can't be calm and happy. Like a mental rumination, I review again, 'where' everything is in place, almost intact. Not more than a few minutes have passed. 'Here' my body is healthy, and nature is incredibly beautiful. As if you are in a place you have dreamed of traveling to, without having to worry about visas, tickets, flights, and money, thrown into one of your dreams. A pleasant foggy morning in the middle of a calm lake, a glass of hot sweet tea in one hand and bread in the other.

I should have been ecstatic, that's right, but I don't feel happy. I had never been caught in my fantasies, that is, my fantasies were never so 'tangible' except in my dreams. And even then, I was not aware that I was dreaming. This is a completely new and unknown situation. A fantasy that is as tangible as my dreams, but unlike my dreams, I am aware that it is imaginary. I have never been in such a state. It is natural to be afraid of this utterly unknown situation, and fear is the biggest obstacle to happiness. Fear and happiness cannot be contained in the same mind at the same time. That is why I am not happy even though I should be.

I recall the words of the shaman. He said that when the story is 'over' I would go back. How should my story end here? For example, if I jump into the lake and drown and die, then my story will end and I would return to real life. Or, on the contrary, if my ethereal body dies here, my physical body will also die there in the middle of the trance state, next to the fire, near the middle of a shamanic ceremony that I didn't believe in?

I don't know! I look at the surface of the lake and think about jumping, a moment of courage is all I need — just jump. Then it will all end. You will shuffle for a few minutes, swallow water, feel suffocated, and then I will probably return to where I originally belonged. I don't know exactly what the experience of drowning is like, but I don't think it would take more than a few minutes. After that, I will be
myself and t

I stare hesitantly at the surface of the lake. The tea has got cold, my hands are dry, and my body is frozen. I just need to muster the courage to leap.

Chapter Five- Che Guevara

My attempt to use intuition did not yield a plausible result. I guessed that Maryam's problem was related to relationships, but this guess had nothing to do with intuition, inspiration, and enlightenment. It was a rational assumption. Maryam was a young woman, and most women about her age and in her cultural and social class, consulted me about their romantic life, so this was only a logical conclusion.

1. Maryam is a young middle-class urban woman.
2. Most middle-class young women who have come to me asked for advice on problems in their relationships.
3. Maryam probably has a problem in her relationships.

This intellectual deduction does not require any intuition or a third eye. The therapist can make correct guesses and conclusions by critical thinking, but the problem is how far these principles can help the therapist. I must find out as I continue the analysis.

Maryam and Fereydoun arrived. I had invited them to my house. This has already been practised by 'Milton Erickson,' an American psychiatrist in Phoenix, Arizona, hence proving that accepting clients at home is not so deconstructive and unorthodox. Of course, from my point of view, but maybe many of my colleagues consider it a violation of 'the principles.'

Erickson's name appears in '*Kaplan and Sadok's* comprehensive textbook of psychiatry, which is the official reference for specialized psychiatry education. Many people, such as Sidney Rosen, Jay Lee, Richard Bandler, and John Grinder, have cited his articles. Therefore, in my opinion, accepting clients at home is not a violation of professional principles. Since I stopped going to the office, I occasionally see clients who can get a 'yes' from me at my classes or in a coffee shop, and if there are no customary cultural restrictions, I see some of them at home. Since Maryam was scheduled to come to the therapy sessions with Fereydoun, her presence in my house did not conflict with the principles of society.

Fereydoun had come to my house for a party last year, and I had seen Maryam for the first time in his villa, so in my opinion, these visits at home did not conflict with therapeutic structures. The future will show whether my arguments are correct or not. I will come to the conclusion that I should have been more bound to 'contracts.' Those big mistakes that Maryam assumed about me during the first session might have been the result of these risky behaviours. I have to list the blunders in my life and see which element in my personality or which repetitive pattern in my behaviour led to those blunders. Was I still repeating those patterns?

Maryam and Fereydoun arrive with a box of assorted chocolates. I welcome them into my house. The big painting of 'Che Guevara' that I have put on the wall makes Maryam happy, and she takes a photo with it. Like me, Maryam loves Che's lifestyle. A guerrilla life, fighting for justice, and to sacrifice for freedom, Freedom from the shackles of institutions and illegitimate powers. From Carol Pearson's point of view, Maryam and I are both within the framework of the archetypes of 'warrior' and 'destroyer' that's why we are fascinated by Che, and wish that our lives would be like his life. In addition, this 'shared fascination' provides me not only with a view of Maryam, but also paints a view of our therapeutic space.

1. The similarity between us, makes it easier for me to communicate with her. We understand each other quickly, so we don't need to force each other to understand things, 'She sees what I know; she knows what I see!'
2. Our similarity makes me blind to Maryam's 'blind spot' because her blind spot is also mine. The healing process may

become a mutual affirmation. I give her a 'well done' card, and she gives me one for actions and beliefs that, from the point of view of another observer (not caught in the Che Guevara model), is nothing but a repeated gross mistake!
3. Maybe this awareness can help me see my own mistakes more clearly because they are similar to her mistakes instead of ignoring my own errors of judgment. Perhaps this could be an example of what Carl Gustav Jung said, 'In every treatment, two people are challenged, the therapist and the client.' Maybe Maryam's therapy leads to my own therapy process. Maybe both of us would heal, maybe one of us, maybe none of us. Also, it is possible that both of us would get worse. I am going through all possible scenarios!
4. I had coffee, Maryam sipped on her tea, and Fereydoun had some green tea. We start with Maryam reviewing her past romantic relationship. Many years ago, after a short session, Maryam fell in love with Mehrdad. She called him on the same day and asked, 'Is there anyone present in your emotional life?' And because 'no one was present,' the relationship between Maryam and Mehrdad begins. A relationship full of tension and pressure because Mehrdad lost his parents in an accident when he was a teenager, and now he lives isolated and withdrawn, suffering from serious psychological injuries.

For years, Maryam's efforts to get Mehrdad out of his moldy shelter remained fruitless. To the extent that many times they contemplate committing suicide together, a bloody ending to a turbulent love, purification, and baptism for a mistake! The archetype of the 'warrior-destroyer' is also presenting itself in Maryam's love. Her love has been 'running in a minefield,' and now, at the end of a war that did not lead to victory, the only testimony that can turn it into a spiritual victory is martyrdom. But suddenly, the scenario changes. Maryam's marriage proposal to Mehrdad (perhaps as the last chance to win) brings him out of the 'psychotic asylum' and he returns to 'life.'

Now, while Maryam should be full of joy and happiness from this 'miracle,' she hesitated whether to stick to her promise or break the marriage arrangement. She has been postponing the ceremony for several months. Being afraid that disrupting Mehrdad's routine will lead him to a more dangerous place than his moldy shelter. On the other hand, she is worried that after marrying Mehrdad when her passion for love has subsided, she would commit an affair of the mind; living with Mehrdad but thinking of someone else!

Chapter Six-Dream Analysis

The shaman said whenever my story ends in 'here,' I will return 'there,' to the world where I truly belong. Why did I think that jumping into the water would end my story? Maybe he meant that whenever you have learned the lesson you needed from this experience, you will return from the inner journey. I have to see what lesson this mental journey has for me and why I was thrown into this fantasy. Perhaps the best way is to analyze this fantasy in the same way Freud taught in his book 'The Interpretation of Dreams,' that is, to break the dream into its constituent parts and 'free association' about each part to create associations. After that, the connection between these associations should be discovered to show the meaning of the whole.

I do not have a pen and paper, so I have to do this mentally. I review the components of the fantasy in my mind, lake, heavy rain, umbrella, rowing girl, boat, oars, huts, The isle movie, loneliness, oil stove, kettle, tea, bread, apple, sugar, loneliness, thick morning mist, and fear of drowning. I think I have identified the main elements. Now I should see what personal unconscious themes each of these 'visual elements' contain for me.

Therefore, I will freely associate each of these elements,

** Lake, femininity, silence, swimming, calmness, coolness, depth, circle.

**Heavy rain, washing, baptism, bath, anger, sky, earth, the memory of Yokohama.

**Umbrella, protection, hide, camouflage, sun, rain, sea, rescue.

** Boat girl, silence, femininity, sex, anima, look.

**Boat, suspension, hanging, toppling, sinking, floating, globe.

** Oar, phallus, sword, dagger, tear, plunge, advance.

** Huts, refuge, shelter, sleep, exhaustion, asylum, relaxation.

** The isle movie, Zen, Buddhism, Kim Ki-duk, Spring, Summer, Autumn, winter and spring again, Korea, Japan, meditation, reincarnation.

** Solitude, silence, introspection, knowledge, relaxation, awareness of the mind.

**Oil stove, fire, heat, food, cooking, light, oil, match, Prometheus.

** Kettle, cooking, drinking, boiling, safety.

** Tea, habit, relaxation, grandfather, samovar, reception, guest.

**Bread, Give us our bread today (prayer), God, Marx, poverty, discrimination.

**Apple, Love, Sohrab, Aphrodite, forbidden fruit, Garden of Eden.

** Sugar, diabetes, insulin, disease, diet, neuropathy, disability.

** Thick fog in the morning, Chiang Mai city, traveling with elephants, beauty, nature, paradise, humidity.

** Fear of drowning, childhood, death, separation from mother, Caspian Sea, waves, pulling rug from under my feet, suffocation.

Now I have to put these words together like pieces of a puzzle to reach a composite and coherent picture. In this journey, my connection with the anima (spirituality-oneness-acceptance) is supposed to be established. I have to achieve oneness and peace with my inner femininity. I have developed an excess of masculinity (rush-speed-movement-control), and the disease (diabetes-incapacitating neuropathy) is my body's reaction to the excessive masculinity. I have to meditate, pray, and lead my life at a slower pace, moment by moment, like a Japanese tea ceremony.

I suddenly come out of sleep/trance/fantasy. We are sitting around the fire. It is night. The last flames are dying down. The red-orange colour covers the beauty of some firewood, while the rest of the firewood is extinguished. The shaman's assistant still occasionally beats the tambourine. But the shaman puts the bell on the ground and pours tea. The first sip of tea burns my throat. Surely, I'm back from my inner journey.

Chapter Seven-Rubber Band

The fact that Maryam was familiar with drama and literature encouraged me to use drama and story techniques in her therapy. In each session, I asked her to play the role of a character other than herself who goes to a psychiatrist and talks about her life. I wanted to bypass the 'resistance.' When people talk about themselves, they worry about the judgment of the audience, even if that audience is their therapist. Then they start to omit and modify what they have in their heart until they create a narrative that they see themselves as acceptable, then this 'narrative' becomes their 'identity,' that is, we see ourselves as we wish others to see us. We are recreated in our creation; the offspring of our creations.

This is akin to the theme of the 'dialectic of self-consciousness' discussed in Hegel's philosophy and Lacan's psychology. But when clients are going to weave a story or play someone else's role, that dynamic changes. They don't feel the responsibility of a hero's life on their shoulders. As a result, they speak more freely, and their thinking patterns are more easily discovered.

In one of the stories, Maryam played the role of a southern woman. A woman with three teenage boys who are busy from morning till night, cleaning, cooking, and housekeeping, she is crippled by fatigue, stress, and the pressure of life. That woman was beaten by her husband, a motorcycle mechanic, but she loves her husband.

With this story, Maryam traveled to the neighbourhoods where she once lived. This story opened her grievance about those years. She talked about life among people where poverty, addiction, and prostitution were a big part of their daily life. As a teenage girl, growing up in such conditions, she had experienced beatings and sexual harassment many times, and it happened that without further probing, she spontaneously talked about those big wounds honestly and without a filter.

In another story, Maryam described the land of her dreams, Paris. This time, Maryam had the same life that she would have had if the world revolved around kindness and love. She had studied philosophy and music, was married to an educated and scholarly husband, and their life was spent in theatres, concerts, and academies in Paris. This story revealed her regrets and dreams.

By putting together, the wounds and regrets from Maryam's stories, I pieced together the pieces of the puzzle and understood why Maryam, despite relatively acceptable conditions in her life today, was full of anger and anxiety. Is it possible to say to the wounds and sigh, 'Shut up and begone?'

Maryam was stuck between two worlds, the world she came from and the world she thought she deserved. Based on the standards of the world, she was moving forward and shining on the red carpet, but based on the world she came from, she felt guilty about her shining victory. She thought she had betrayed the neighbourhood she came from if drown in the glory of awards and celebrations, so whenever her achievements seemed adequate, her guilt pulled her back to his origin like a rubber band.

She then returned to those who were drowned in psychological and social wounds and tried to pay for her contribution to this world. But this duality would not let her go, the game of the savior/victim, always reached the limit, she missed the awards and shining on the stage, and she was tired of the continuation of this endless nursing role and wanted to escape. This was exactly the point where she was with Mehrdad.

Chapter Eight- Damascus

I think about my 'big gaffe.' I ponder over the similarity between Maryam and my fascination with Che Guevara. I review the pathway of my life and the mysterious and hidden compulsions in my life choices. I contemplate Maryam getting stuck between the downtown poor suburbs and Champs Élysées in Paris, and ask myself, 'Which two worlds are you torn between?'

I go to sleep with this question and travel to Damascus in my sleep – the same dreamlike neighbourhoods of old Damascus that evoke the tales of *'The thousand and one nights'*. Legends in which we can find a magic lamp in the closet, and if you search the dark underground corridors of the house, you would find a dirt-covered carpet rolled up in the bottom of a big green wooden box, which must be Solomon's flying carpet.

I enter the Bab Toma neighbourhood from the eastern door and walk down the narrow 'Hananieh' street towards the church. The weather is neither cold nor hot, it is as it should be. The streets are neither crowded nor lonely, they are as they should be. On the right side, there are houses with courtyards in front of the rooms, and on the left side are old two-story mansions with beautiful Arabic windows, the crescent being the most prominent visual element of them.

The mansions feature small balconies where refreshing vases are beautifully arranged. The high walls of the mansions awaken the feeling that you are drowning little by little in the alleys and going deeper in. When I go a little further, on the right side, I see a small prayer hall with stone walls, the size of a small room. The space inside the prayer hall is cold, maybe because of the stone walls, and it is dark because there are no windows. It is wintertime and an old servant of the prayer hall has stretched out his legs on the platform next to the entrance door and thrown a blanket over his legs. He has turned on a small electric heater to warm up his feet.

I light a candle at the altar and kneel, clasping my hands together to pray, but what kind of prayer? I do not know! I haven't prayed for years, but on all my tourist trips, I have visited temples, mosques, and churches! At this moment, someone puts a hand on my shoulder. I turn and look – a tall man in a hooded Arab attire, one of those worn by Moroccans, is standing next to me. He doesn't seem familiar in the darkness of the prayer hall. We greet each other and shake hands. Now I recognise him, it's Yunus. I met him in Medina, in Masjid al-Nabi and in the midday prayer line, he was sitting to my right. They hadn't called the call to prayer yet, and I was reading the Quran. When I closed the Quran and kissed it, he asked, 'Do you know what word is in the middle of the Quran?'

I did not know. He answered, 'Waliltaf,' which means 'One should be gentle.'

And now Yunus is standing next to me, this time in Damascus in Orthodox prayer halls on Hananiyah Street. Next, I am walking in the streets with Yunus, as if it is a dinner invitation and he has invited me to his friend's house. Yaqub, the host, is an Assyrian from Syria. Yaqoob's house is one of the houses depicted in *'One Thousand and One Nights'*. We walk inside the corridor and reach a large yard with a hexagonal pond in the middle. The yard is swept, and the smell of damp soil is perfused in the air. The air is cold after the sunset, and because of the steam in the room, it is blurry behind the windows. The table is spread, and we eat Arabic rice full of spices, and we hear about Yaqub's memories of his marriage.

Twenty years later, he still wanted to know what I think about putting a spell on the groom so that he accepts all the conditions of the bride's family. He thinks that such a spell had befallen him that he had accepted all the conditions immediately. I don't know what to say, so I try to change the topic, but it is important for him to know my opinion. I say that if your mother-in-law knew how to put a spell on you, she would have done it in such a way that after twenty years, you would not regret accepting their conditions. He laughs, but I think he is still stuck to his belief.

Now I see myself in Hamidiyeh market, in Yaqub's store; he was a spice seller. The prickling smell of spices fills the room, the shelves are filled with all kinds of spices and bottles of spirits. Yaqub pours Arabic coffee into small cups and places the dried date plate in front of me. His peasant puts a long Arabic hookah in front of us, and the smell of aromatic tobacco adds to the smell of Arabic spices and perfume. The hookah rings are floating in the air. The market is busy and crowded, and the babel of the vendors erupts from every corner.

Chapter Nine-The Aftermath

Three years have passed since the last session with Maryam. Fereydon calls to tell me that Maryam has come to Iran and wants to see me. This time we are session in a coffee shop in Yousef Abad (a suburb in Tehran). The man behind the counter knows Maryam and wants to take a selfie with her, probably for his Instagram. Maryam abruptly refuses. They haven't brought the coffee yet, when the tears slowly start to flow from her saddened eyes.

Three years ago, after three sessions of therapy, Maryam decided that she had as many sessions as necessary and did not continue the sessions. This is not a rare scenario, in fact, most of my clients, other than those who were undergoing drug treatment, would come to a conclusion after a few sessions that they had achieved what they needed and left. Until a few years later, sometimes ten years later, they return, sometimes with a new story and sometimes with a repetition of the previous story but in a new form.

Maryam had broken off her relationship with Mehrdad three years ago, and fortunately, Mehrdad had neither committed suicide nor returned to addiction. However, today, she was not going to talk about Mehrdad and her relationship with him, as if that story was a distant memory.

During these years, Maryam experienced another exciting story. Although this story had a completely different shell, it still showed the back and forth between the two worlds, just like a rubber band. This time, Maryam has been abandoned, and now she was heartbroken, a mixture of longing and regret, astonishment and feeling of rejection. There is no time for analysis right now, as I have to help Maryam manage her emotions and get back to her life. We will get to the depth of her repetitive patterns, maybe some other time, when the time is right.

About the Author

Born on the 26th of October in Zabul (Sistan), I spent my childhood in the south of Khorasan and my adolescence in Mashhad. When I was nine years old, the revolution of 1979 occurred in Iran, and our generation has had the chance to witness a moving era, and many of their beliefs have been challenged. Many of the 'good' became 'bad' and vice versa, and the names of the streets were changed many times. Our generation 'witnessed' the war. Some of my friends and classmates were killed on the battlefield. Their funeral introduced me to the concept of 'death' at a young age.

At the end of the eight-year war, I entered Zahedan Medical School in the fall of 1989. I have been practicing medicine since 1998. In addition to my medical studies, I was involved in cultural studies (i.e., history, religion, political science) and social activities throughout my undergraduate degree. When I was nineteen, I wrote my first book, 'The Puzzle of Time' about Einstein`s relativity theory, and a contribution to understanding religious texts- it was published in 1994.

After reading the works of the famous Swiss psychiatrist Carl Gustav Jung, I entered the realm of psychiatry. In the fall of 1998, I started my psychiatry course at Mashhad University of Medical Sciences. In 2001, I passed the specialty board of psychiatry and became a member of the faculty of Medicine at Mashhad University. Entering the realm of psychiatry has deepened the challenges that the 'Social-Political transition' had created for me. The field of psychiatry and psychoanalysis is my favorite as it challenges the most basic concepts of the human mind. There are fewer ones to enter this domain, with their 'belief system' remaining unchanged.

Personally, I am more interested in mystical views, but the data analysis results have forced me to change the content of my works and abandon my deep nostalgia- sometimes the right path is the hardest way!

Mohammad Reza Sargolzaee

MEDICAL EDUCATION

1988- 1995, Doctor of medicine degree from Zahedan University of Medical Sciences

PSYCHIATRIC TRAINING

1997 – 2000, Psychiatric residency training at Mashad University of Medical Sciences

EMPLOYMENT HISTORY

2014 – Present, Therapist and Educator, Alcoholism Clinic, Iranian Center For Addiction Studies (INCAS), Tehran, Iran.

2001- Now, Lecturer in Psychotherapy, Iranian Scientific Society of Clinical Hypnosis (ISSCH), Tehran, Iran.

2000 – 2003, Assistant Professor, Department of Psychiatry, Mashad University of Medical Sciences, Iran.

1997 – 2000, Senior Specialist, Addition clinic (Multi – disciplinary approach), Welfare Organization, Mashad, Iran.

1997- 2000, Resident of Psychiatry, Psychiatry Researcher, Shafa Psychiatry Hospital, Mashad, Iran.

1995-1997, General Practitioner / Medical Researcher, BOO-ALI Hospital, Zahedan, Iran.

1993-1995, Medical Intern / medical researcher, Khatam-Al-Anbia General Hospital, Zahedan, Iran.

PUBLICATIONS

BOOKS

1. Sargolzaee M.R (1993), The Mystery of Time, Sepah Publication.

2. Sargolzaee M.R and Keikhaee N. (1994), MCQ (Multiple Choice Questions) of Pediatrics. (translation)

3. Sargolzaee M.R and Zohravi T. (1999), Psychiatric Drugs, Gol-Aftab Publication, (translation)

4. Sargolzaee M.R (2000), When You Must Go To A Psychiatrist, Mashad University Press.

5. Sargolzaee M.R (2000), The Successful Management of Substance Dependence, Mashad University Press. (Winner of the President's prize)

6. Sargolzaee M.R and Azarpazhooh H (2002), OCD, Ferdowsi University Press, (translation)

7. Sargolzaee M.R (2002), THE WAY (psychotherapy of addiction), Welfare Organization Publications

8- Sargolzaee M R(2003), I don't want This (about problem-solving), Marandiz Publication

9- Sargolzaee M R(2003), Life, thinking, and no more (about critical Thinking), Marandiz Publication

10-Sargolzaee M R(2003), The Love Stories (about the romantic relationship and rationality), Marandiz Publication
11- Sargolzaee M R(2003), The letters to the Sky (about spirituality), Marandiz Publication

12- Sargolzaee M R(2003), 10 questions, no answers (about philosophy), Marandiz Publication

13- Sargolzaee M R(2005), Healthy Personality, Qatre Publication

14-Sargolzaee M R(2005), Addiction, causality and treatment,, Qatre Publication

15- Sargolzaee M R(2005), the note book of a psychiatrist,, Qatre Publication

16- Sargolzaee M R(2003), the Life lessons from Mathnavi of Mevlana, Marandiz Publication

17- Sargolzaee M R(2003), 1001 nights between sleep and awakening (about the mystical experience), Marandiz Publication

18-Sargolzaee M (2003)R, 1,2,3 move! (about life skills), Marandiz Publication

19- Sargolzaee M R(2011) , Life and Freedom, Fariwar Publication

20-Sargolzaee M R(2012), for the people of today (about community psychology of Iranian people), Bahaare-sabz Publication

21- Sargolzaee M R (2014), Human-Philosophy-Mysticism, Bahaare-Sabz Publication,

22- sargolzaee M R (2015) , Life Skills for Adolescents, bahaare-Sabz Publication

PAPERS

1. Sargolzaee, M.R., Keikhaee N., Sargolzaee S. (1995), HBV Contamination in the Dentistry Instruments, the Journal of Students & Research, Shiraz University of Medical Sciences, 9(3), 22-26

2. Sargolzaee, M.R.(1993), Abdominal Masses in the Children, Iranian Congress of Pediatric New Findings, Yazd University of Medical Sciences, Abstract book

3. Sargolzaee, M.R. & Keikhaee N. (1994), the Study of the Sensitivity of the Microorganisms in the Urine Cultures, Iranian Congress of Microbiology, Yazd University of Medical Sciences, Abstract book

4. Abdollahian E., Sargolzaee M.R. and Ekhteraee M.(1998), the Approach to a Patient with Conversion Symptoms, NAVID Journal, Mashad University of Medical Sciences, 14, 15-19

5. Sargolzaee, M.R . and Salimi M. (1998); the Study of the Administration of Psychotropic Drugs by the General Practitioners of Khorasan, the Iranian Congress of Psychopharmacology, Isfahan University of Medical Sciences, Abstract book

6. Sargolzaee, M.R . (1999), the Pathophysiology of Addiction, the Congress of the Treatment of Addiction, Birjand University of Medical Sciences, Abstract book

7. Sargolzaee, M.R. & Keikhaee N. (1999), Dysmenorrhea and Sport in Woman, Journal of Yasuj University of Medical Sciences, 12 (3), 52 – 56

8. Sargolzaee, M.R.(1999), the Brief Psychotherapies for Substance Dependence, the Congress of Health Strategies for Addiction, Zahedan University of Medical sciences, Abstract book

9. Sargolzaee, M.R. (2000), Stress and Dysmenorrhea, 6th World Congress on ' Innovations in Psychiatry – 2000, 'London University, Abstract book

10. Abdollahian E and Sargolzaee, M.R. (2000), the prevalence of depression and the effect of Psychosocial factors in the students, 6th World Congress on '(Innovations in Psychiatry-2000),' London University, abstract book

11. Sargolzaee, M.R. (2000), Sexual dysfunction after opioid withdrawal, Navid Journal, Mashad University of Medical sciences, 19, 25 – 27

12. Sargolzaee, M.R. (2000), psychotherapy and prosody, 2nd Iranian congress of music Therapy, Tehran University of medical sciences, abstract book

13. Sargolzaee, M.R., Abdollahian E and Erfanian A. (2000), the study of Dynamics of the children of opioid-dependent parents based on

CAT, 4th Iranian seminar on children and adolescents mental Health, Zanjan university of medical sciences, Abstract Book

14. Abdollahian E. and Sargolzaee M.R. (2000), the correlation between positive waves in EEG and psychiatric disorders in the children and Adolescents, Journal of Mashad university of Medical sciences, 67,89-94

15. Abdollahian E., Nozadi Gh. and Sargolzaee M.R. (2000), the economic burden of Depressive Disorders, the Journal of psychiatry and clinical psychology (Andishe – va – Raftar), 6(1), 20 – 25

16. Sargolzaee M.R. and Fayyazi M.R. (2000), Psychotherapy and the Economy of the Treatment, the Journal of Health (Reza Behzistan), 17, 30 – 35

17. Sargolzaee M.R. (2000), the Motivation for substance abuse, the Iranian congress of socio-Cultural causes of Addiction, Tehran culture office, Abstract book

18. Sargolzaee, M.R. and Moharreri F (2000), Detoxification, the Journal of Khorasan social security Organization, 3, 16-19

19. Behdani, F. , Sargolzaee M.R. and Ghorbani E (2000), the correlation between life style and Depression and Anxiety in the students, the journal of Sabzewar school of medicine, 2, 27 – 38

20. Sargolzaee M.R. , Karimi Sh. and Fayyazi M.R. (2000), the efficacy of calcium-D tablets on the reduction of the symptoms of withdrawal of opioids, the journal of Sabzewar school of medicine,4, 9 – 14

21. Sargolzaee, M.R. , Moharreri F. , Arshadi H.R. et al. (2001), Depression and Sexual Dysfunction in the Infertile, Medical journal of reproduction and infertility, 8(2) ,46-52

22. Sargolzaee,M.R. , Fayyazi M.R., Aghaee M. et al. (2001), the study of the attitudes and level of information of non – psychiatrist physicians about psychiatry, the international congress of new commitments for psychiatrists, WPA, Madrid, abstract book

23. Sargolzaee, M.R. , Behdani F., Ghorbani E. (2001), the study of Correlation between time spent in Religious Activities and

Depression, Anxiety and Substance Abuse in the students, the International Congress of new commitments for psychiatrists, WPA, Madrid, abstract book

24. Sargolzaee M.R. and Zohravi T.(2001), Study of Sensitivity, Specifily and effectivity of morphine check Kits for diagnosis of Narcotic use, Journal of Legal Medicine of Islamic Republic of Iran, 23, 19 – 28

25. Toofani H. and Sargolzaee M.R. (2001), Clozapine and Neuroleptic Malignant Syndrome, Medical Journal of Mashad University of Medical Sciences, 44 (73), 137 – 140

26. Sargolzaee M.R. (2002), Neurolinguistic programming in the treatment of phobia, Iranian congress of psychiatric new findings, Tehran university of medical sciences, abstract book

27. Sargolzaee M.R. (2002), Nutritional habits in Iranian pioid dependents, Eating disorders conference 2002, Austria, Abstract book.

28. Social Welfare Fall 2003; 3(9),294-283. the case study of narcotic drug abuse abundance and its relationship to Mashhad medical student's personal and family condition, Sargolzaee M.R., Balali M., Azad R., Ardekani M.R., Samari A.A.

29. Sargolzaei, MR. Samari, AA. Keykhany, AA (2003) Neuro-cognitive behavioral therapy in test anxiety control, Journal of mental health, fifth issue, in spring and summer (1382) Number seventeenth and eighteenth, Pp.42 -34.

30. Stereological Volumetry of Cerebral Hemispheres and Lateral Ventricles Using MRI in Schizophrenia Subtypes, H Haghir, M R Sargolzaee, J Jalal Shokouhi, M T Shakeri, Iranian Journal of Radiology 2004; 2(1-2),34-41

31. Relationship between marital satisfaction during Pregnancy and Postpartum Depression (PPD). F. Kiani, T. Khadivzadeh, M. R. Sargolzaee, H. Behnam, Iranian Journal of Obstetrics, Gynecology and Infertility 2010;13(5), 37-44.

32. Lipid profile comparison between opium addicts and non-addicts. S. S. Fatemi, M. Hasanzadeh, A. Arghami, M. R. Sargolzaee, Journal of Tehran University Heart Center 2008;3(3), 169-172.

33. Gender dimorphism in the DAT1-67 T-allele homozygosity and predisposition to bipolar disorder. M. Ohadi, M. R. Keikhaee, A. Javanbakht, M. R. Sargolzaee, M. Robabeh, H. Najmabadi, Brain Research 2007;1144(), 142-145.

34. Gender dimorphism in the DAT1 – 67 T-allele homozygosity and predisposition to bipolar disorder. M. Ohadi, M. R. Keikhaee, A. Javanbakht, M. R. Sargolzaee, M. Robabeh, H. Najmabadi, Brain Research 2007;1144(1), 142-145.

35. Association between interleukin-10 promoter polymorphisms and schizophrenia in the Iranian population. Z. Sabouri, S. N. Bajestan, H. Takashima, M. R. Sargolzaee, M. N. Bajestan, R. Farid, K. Arimura, A. Sano, M. Osame, Journal of Neuroimmunology 2006;178(), 182-182.

36. Study of the efficacy of fluoxetine and clomipramine in the treatment of premature ejaculation after opioid detoxification. E. Abdollahian, A. Javanbakht, K. Javidi, A. A. Samari, M. Shakiba, M. R. Sargolzaee, American Journal on Addictions 2006;15(1), 100-104.

37. Association of AKT1 haplotype with the risk of schizophrenia in the Iranian population. S. N. Bajestan, A. H. Sabouri, M. Nakamura, H. Takashima, M. R. Keikhaee, F. Behdani, M. R. Fayyazi, M. R. Sargolzaee, M. N. Bajestan, Z. Sabouri, E. Khayami, S. Haghighi, S. B. Hashemi, N. Eiraku, H. Tufani, H. Najmabadi, K. Arimura, A. Sano, M. Osame, American Journal of Medical Genetics Part B-Neuropsychiatric Genetics 2006;141B(4), 383-386.

38. Association of AKT1 haplotype with the risk of schizophrenia in the Iranian population. S. N. Bajestan, A. H. Sabouri, M. Nakamura, H. Takashima, M. R. Keikhaee, F. Behdani, M. R. Fayyazi, M. R. Sargolzaee, M. N. Bajestan, Z. Sabouri, E. Khayami, S. Haghighi, S. B. Hashemi, N. Eiraku, H. Tufani, H. Najmabadi, K. Arimura, A. Sano, M. Osame, American Journal of Medical Genetics, Part B, Neuropsychiatric Genetics 2006;141(4), 383-386.

39. Association of AKTI haplotypes with the risk of schizophrenia in the Iranian population. S. N. Bajestan, M. Nakamura, M. R. Keikhaee, M. R. Sargolzaee, M. N. Bajestan, Z. Sabouri, A. Sano, M. Osame, Journal of the Neurological Sciences 2005;238(), S339-S339.

40. Association analysis of the dopamine transporter (DAT1)-67A/T polymorphism in bipolar disorder. M. R. Keikhaee, F. Fadai, M. R. Sargolzaee, A. Javanbakht, H. Najmabadi, M. Ohadi, American Journal of Medical Genetics Part B-Neuropsychiatric Genetics 2005;135B(1), 47-49.

41. Clinical subtypes of OCD and importance of early detection of psychotic pseudo-OCD. M. R. Sargolzaee, Schizophrenia Research 2004;70(1), 114-114.

42. Effects of desmopressin (DDAVP) on memory impairment following electroconvulsive therapy. M. R. Sargolzaee, E. Abdollahian, M. Hajzade, M. D. Mohebbi, International Journal of Psychophysiology 2004;54(1-2), 112-112.

43. The comparison of the efficacy of citrus fragrance and fluoxetine in the treatment of major depressive disorder. M. R. Sargolzaee, A. A. Samari, M. R. F. Bordbar, International Journal of Psychophysiology 2004;54(1-2), 111-112.

44. Effects of desmopressin (DDAVP) on memory impairment following electroconvulsive therapy (ECT). E. Abdollahian, M. R. Sargolzaee, M. Hajzade, M. D. Mohebbi, A. Javanbakht, Acta Neuropsychiatrica 2004;16(3), 130-137.

45. Gender dimorphism in the DAT1-67 T-allele homozygosity and predisposition to bipolar disorder. M. Ohadi, M. R. Keikhaee, A. Javanbakht, M. R. Sargolzaee, M. Robabeh, H. Najmabadi, Brain Research 2007;(1144), 142-145.

46. Association of AKT1 haplotype with the risk of schizophrenia in the Iranian population. S. N. Bajestan, A. H. Sabouri, M. Nakamura, H. Takashima, M. R. Keikhaee, F. Behdani, M. R. Fayyazi, M. R. Sargolzaee, M. N. Bajestan, Z. Sabouri, E. Khayami, S. Haghighi, S. B. Hashemi, N. Eiraku, H. Tufani, H. Najmabadi, K. Arimura, A. Sano, M.

Osame, American Journal of Medical Genetics Part B-Neuropsychiatric Genetics 2006;4(141B), 383-386.

47. Association analysis of the dopamine transporter (DAT1)-67A/T polymorphism in bipolar disorder. M. R. Keikhaee, F. Fadai, M. R. Sargolzaee, A. Javanbakht, H. Najmabadi, M. Ohadi, American Journal of Medical Genetics Part B-Neuropsychiatric Genetics 2005;1(135B), 47-49.

48. Association of AKTI haplotypes with the risk of schizophrenia in the Iranian population. S. N. Bajestan, M. Nakamura, M. R. Keikhaee, M. R. Sargolzaee, M. N. Bajestan, Z. Sabouri, A. Sano, M. Osame, Journal of the Neurological Sciences 2005;(238), S339-S339.

www.ingramcontent.com/pod-product-compliance
Lightning Source LLC
Chambersburg PA
CBHW050330220526
45465CB00012B/397